W9-ATA-032

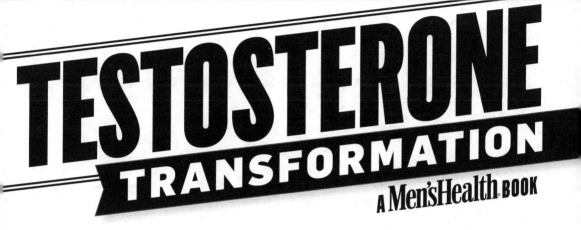

TESTOSTERONE TRANSFORMATION

A Men'sHealth BOOK

LOSE BELLY FAT, BUILD MUSCLE & BOOST SEXUAL VITALITY

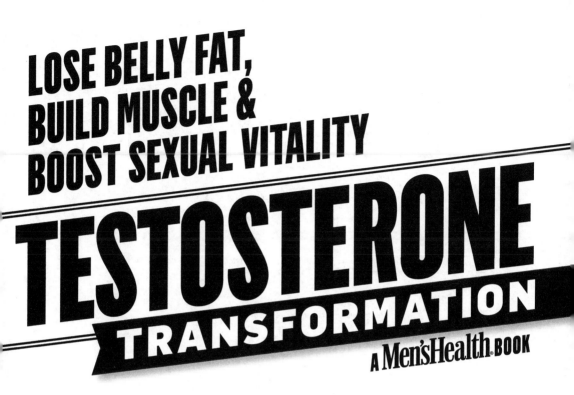

TESTOSTERONE TRANSFORMATION

A Men'sHealth BOOK

BY **MYATT MURPHY**, C.S.C.S.

RODALE.

Book design by Mike Smith
Photographs by Thomas MacDonald
Cover photograph by Scott McDermott

Library of Congress Cataloging-in-Publication Data

Murphy, Myatt.
Testosterone transformation : lose belly fat, build muscle, & boost sexual vitality / Myatt Murphy.
p. cm.
ISBN 978-1-60961-774-5 (hardcover)
1. Men—Health and hygiene. 2. Testosterone—Physiological effect.
I. Title.
RA777.8.M87 2012
613'.0423—dc23
ISBN-13: 978-1-60961-774-5

2 4 6 8 10 9 7 5 3   hardcover

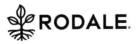

DEDICATION

To Beth:
For always being patient—and being perfect in every way.

CONTENTS

ACKNOWLEDGEMENTS

When I was hired as a staff editor by *Men's Health* magazine in 1993, I wasn't looking to forge a career as a writer—I was simply there to bide enough time to decide what my next step in life might be.

I never fully understood how lucky I was back then to be there during the magazine's formative years. Over time, I came to realize that I had worked side-by-side with individuals who to this day continue to be some of the most innovative and dedicated editors and visionaries in publishing.

Testosterone Transformation is the fourth book I've written for *Men's Health*— *The Body You Want in the Time You Have, Men's Health's Gym Bible,* and *Men's Health Ultimate Dumbbell Guide* being the other three—but it's the first that has allowed me to reconnect with three members of that original team: *Men's Health* Editor-in-Chief David Zinczenko; Stephen Perrine, acting publisher of Rodale Books; and my editor on this book, Jeff Csatari, the most ethical and impassioned editor I've ever known throughout my 17-year career.

To Dave, Steve, and Jeff: I'm very proud (and not surprised) to see how far each of you has come in life, and even prouder to have had the chance to work with you many years ago, and once again on this book. Thank you for pushing me and guiding me when I was too young and green at the time to truly appreciate it.

My sincerest thanks go out to Josh Bryant (the most discerning, yet humble exercise expert I have ever teamed up with) and Tara Gidus (whose infinite knowledge of nutrition always makes me realize how much I wish I knew).

Special thanks to the other key experts who contributed to this book: Mixed Martial Arts strength and conditioning coach superstar Kelly Tekin; multiple-award-winning trainer C.J. Murphy; top endocrinologist Robert J. Saltman, MD; Darryn S. Willoughby, PhD; Cedric Bryant; and Emily Groff (for giving everything her never-miss once-over.)

My heartfelt gratitude goes out to the talented designer of this book, Mike Smith; Design Director George Karabotsos; photographer Thomas MacDonald and his team of Troy Schnyder and Ayla Christman; and the entire Rodale book editorial team, including Debbie McHugh, Chris Krogermeier, Sara Cox, Erin Williams, and Sean Sabo.

And, finally, I wish to thank my dad, Skip. This former Marine taught me the value of fitness and the importance of staying in shape, so that one day I could do the same for you.

MYATT MURPHY

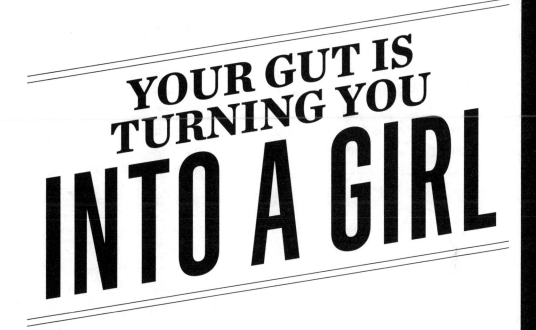

YOUR GUT IS TURNING YOU INTO A GIRL

Trimming your belly is the best route to more testosterone and massive muscle

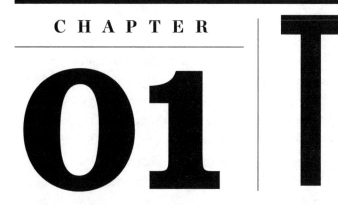

CHAPTER

01

Testosterone. The very mention of the word causes a man's ears to perk up. From our muscles to our manhood, it's the inborn elixir that makes us men.

Testosterone is the very symbol of strength, honor, dominance, self-reliance, sexuality, virility, muscularity, and every other character trait associated with masculinity that men always wish they had more of—even if they already have plenty. It's what determines the hair on our chests, how much muscle pops through our shirts, how much heft we can hoist over our heads, and the strength of our erections. It's what gives a man an edge in competition, whether it's winning the big game, wooing the ladies, or walloping his co-workers in the race for the corner office. Competition, physical skill, size, muscle, and strength are entwined in the concept of masculinity in virtually every culture on earth.

It's safe to assume that there's nothing about testosterone that men don't appreciate or love to hear. Except for one tiny little thing: As you read this, you're turning your personal testosterone spigot in the wrong direction.

Your body is at war with itself, and, unfortunately for you, odds are you're not on the winning side. Testosterone levels in American men have been declining steadily over the past 2 decades, declared a study in the prestigious *Journal of Clinical Endocrinology & Metabolism* a few years back. Typically, testosterone levels in men peak around their late twenties and gradually decline from 30 on. This study, however, showed that 20 years ago 50-year-olds had higher T concentrations than they do today, suggesting that something other than age may be contributing to declines. The researchers reported that the reasons for the decline were unclear but speculated that unmeasured health or environmental factors could be the cause.

Scientists do know that health and lifestyle can exert significant influence on the up-and-down fluctuations of testosterone in the body. Seemingly everything you do—from what you eat and how many hours you sleep to the types of activities and exercises you choose—has either a "promising" or a "punishing" effect on testosterone production. Even seemingly immaterial things that you do or expose yourself to during the course of an average day, such as rooting for unlucky sports teams or reaching for the wrong kind of body soap—can choke off the volume of testosterone that your testicles create. The fact of the matter is this: If you're not happy with how fit and muscular you are or how you're performing in life, it may not be your testicles that are to blame but how you are holding them back from keeping you powerful, primed, and potent.

YOUR BELLY AND YOUR BOYS

I f you're middle-aged, your body's testosterone levels (T-levels) have already begun their slow descent from where they once hovered when you were 18 and too young to appreciate it.

The average guy experiences a gradual decline in testosterone starting around age 30. At age 40, T levels drop by about 2 percent each year. It's a slow, steady, natural tailspin, but as those endocrinology researchers found, that doesn't mean time is the only factor contributing to the dip. Even if you're 24, virile, and officially in the prime of your T-making years, that doesn't mean you're not facing a drop in testosterone right now. Take this simple test: The next time you step out of the shower, before you reach for the towel, stand up straight and look down at your boys. If you can see your testicles, congratulations, Mr. T. But if a big belly is blocking your view, it's likely that your testosterone levels aren't what they could be. Belly fat, my friend, is a testosterone buster.

Being overweight is a serious concern for the average guy for a host of health-related reasons. High blood pressure, coronary heart disease, Type 2 diabetes, cancer, stroke, sleep apnea, respiratory issues, and osteoporosis are just a few of the fun things that being overweight can make you more susceptible to. But even if all those syndromes don't scare you into dropping a few pounds, here's the best reason to look at your belly as the enemy: It's secretly turning you into a girl.

We know what you're thinking: Having excess body fat rounds out a man, making him look more curvaceous than cut and, if he's really unlucky, giving him a pair of man breasts to match. But that's not what we mean when we refer to fat's power to make you girly. Stored body fat, you see, contains aromatase, a nasty little enzyme that's responsible for converting testosterone into estrogen, the main sex hormone in women. What's worse, having extra estrogen floating around your system automatically triggers your body to slow down its production of testosterone. That means the more fat you stockpile, the less testosterone your gonads will give up. It's a vicious cycle: Belly fat means more estrogen and less testosterone, which in turn means additional belly fat.

According to a 2008 epidemiological study of 1,822 men by the New England Research Institutes (NERI), a man's waist circumference is the single strongest predictor of low testosterone levels—even more accurate than age or overall health. Midriff weight, researchers say, also is the strongest predictor of what's called symptomatic androgen deficiency, or AD, a condition marked by low libido, erectile dysfunction, osteoporosis, depression, lethargy, and diminished physical performance.

Another study demonstrated how weight gain accelerates natural age-related declines in testosterone. When researchers at NERI monitored the health of 1,667 men aged 40 to 70 for 15 years, they discovered that men who gained weight were more likely to experience a more rapid drop in their T-levels than men who had not gained weight. In fact, just a 4 to 5 percent increase in body-mass index (BMI)—reflecting roughly 30 pounds of weight gain for the average man—triggered a decline in a man's T-levels equal to aging 10 years.

MUSCLE MASS AFFECTS T, TOO

ompounding the problem of declining testosterone is the natural age-related loss of muscle mass. According to research at the Jean Mayer USDA Human Nutrition Research Center on Aging, at Tufts University, muscle mass begins to decline about 1 to 2 percent a year from age 30 onward. That can amount to between 10 and 16 ounces of muscle each year. Muscle loss contributes to the age-related slowdown in your metabolic rate, which can cause your body to add a pound of fat per year as well.

This is an ounce-for-ounce, pound-for-pound metabolic remodeling that most men never see coming. Even if you maintain your body weight, you could be saying goodbye to what you want to keep (muscle) and hello to what you want to lose (body fat). That swap, which may not be very noticeable from a visual standpoint, could be sending your T-levels down even further.

The good news in all of this is that you can reverse age-related muscle loss and metabolism decline with resistance exercises. In fact, researchers at the Nutrition, Exercise Physiology, and Sarcopenia Laboratory at Tufts proved that it can happen even in people 70 to 89 years old. In a study of 213 volunteers published in *Medicine & Science in Sports & Exercise*, sedentary elderly folks who were put on a home-based progressive strength, balance, and fitness program added muscle, strength, and cardiovascular endurance. Those who improved the most exercised 150 minutes or more per week.

If the elderly can reap those benefits, consider what strength training can do for you. You can pack on muscle, lose your gut, burn calories efficiently—even at rest—and help your body produce optimum levels of the male hormone. That's what the *Testosterone Transformation* is all about.

From this book, you'll understand not only why having plenty of man's greatest hormone is vital for staying strong, muscular, and energetic, but how testosterone is equally responsible for reducing your risk of developing metabolic syndrome, diabetes, heart disease, and other dangerous medical conditions.

You'll learn step by step how to challenge your body with the type of resistance training the pros use—the high-intensity training that torches unwanted body fat while simultaneously forcing your body to release more testosterone than ever before.

You'll discover why eating the right types of foods—especially certain foods that most people believe are unhealthy for you—can trim off the pounds and throw your T-levels into overdrive.

You'll explore how to maximize every minute of your day—from the time you wake up until the time you fall asleep—so that everything you do helps you build a fitter body and live a healthier life.

Best of all, you're going to accomplish all of it in just 12 weeks.

So what are you waiting for? It's time to grab that spigot, turn it in the right direction, and let that testosterone flow.

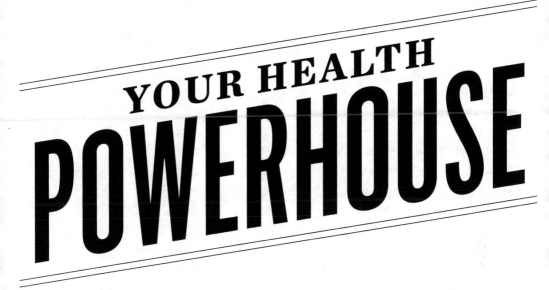

YOUR HEALTH
POWERHOUSE

What more testosterone can do for you

CHAPTER

02

Let's get to know testosterone a little better. Androgenic hormones are what give a guy his guylike characteristics. These male sex hormones act as tiny chemical messengers floating through your system and communicating with specific tissues within your body to control and stimulate their development.

Their main job is keeping your sex drive strong and making sure you're plenty potent to reproduce. However, they also play a vital role in helping your body maintain other "male-based" traits, including body- and facial-hair growth, the lower tone in your voice, and the bone mass that makes up your frame, as well as the muscle that covers it.

Testosterone is one of your body's top androgens, playing a part in everything from controlling how much fat you store to how much overall energy you have throughout the day. "In the simplest sense, people associate testosterone with the genital region, but in a broader sense, like all hormones, it acts everywhere throughout your body—it's even important to overall mental health," says Robert J. Saltman, MD, clinical associate professor in internal medicine and endocrinology at the Washington University School of Medicine, in St. Louis.

One of testosterone's most notable jobs is building lean muscle tissue by allowing your body to increase protein synthesis—the method by which your body repairs and grows muscle after exercise. The hormone also decreases the muscle-protein breakdown that occurs when your body cannibalizes muscle and organ tissue when it goes looking for a source of energy.

Where Does T Come From?

As its name indicates, testosterone is mostly produced by the testicles. However, few guys realize that a tiny amount is also made within the outer portion of the adrenal glands (the adrenal cortex), located on top of the kidneys.

Even though the bulk of your T production takes place down south, it's actually your brain that triggers the process from up above. It starts with your hypothalamus, the part of your brain that's considered its "command center." Responsible for mediating many of your endocrine, autonomic, and behavioral functions—including controlling your body temperature, determining how hungry or thirsty you feel, and even what type of mood you're in—your hypothalamus steers your ship by sending signals via hormones to your pituitary gland, the part of your brain that controls your body's balance of a wide variety of hormones (including testosterone).

The order from brain to balls to brawn goes something like this:

1) When your brain senses the need to produce more testosterone, your hypothalamus (located in the middle of the base of your brain) secretes gonadotropin-releasing hormone (GnRH), which makes its way to the pituitary gland, located in the back of your brain.

2) Your pituitary gland receives that chemical signal from your hypothalamus loud and clear and responds in kind by producing and secreting two specific hormones into your bloodstream: follicle-stimulating hormone (FSH) and luteinizing hormone (LH). Together, these two are called gonadotropins—a dynamic duo that quickly become your T-level's new best friends.

3) These gonadotropins find their way through your bloodstream down to your testicles, where each evokes a different response from your family jewels. FSH reminds your testes to produce more sperm, while LH tells your testes to produce more testosterone by stimulating your Leydig cells (the testosterone-producing cells within each testicle).

4) Your Leydig cells are really the ones working overtime inside your testicles to create plenty of T, a task they pull off by converting cholesterol into testosterone. Your Leydig cells have two options when finding all the cholesterol they need to make that transformation take place: They can either absorb cholesterol from your blood or, if necessary, produce cholesterol themselves.

5) Once testosterone is produced, it is sent back into your bloodstream, where it immediately goes to work stimulating the development of your muscles and bones, your body-fat placement, and other areas.

6) All that extra testosterone gets your brain's attention. If the brain determines that your testes are pumping out too much testosterone, your hypothalamus sends another signal to your pituitary gland to secrete less LH, which in turn lowers how much testosterone your testes will produce.

What's Considered a Normal Level?

The average amount most men have flowing through their veins is between 300 and 1,000 ng/dl (nanograms per deciliter of blood), depending on how old they are. But as I mentioned in Chapter 1, after you hit 40, your body hits back by reducing the amount of testosterone it produces by about 1 to 2 percent each year.

Anything below 300 ng/dl is not only considered low, but it could be an indicator that you're a likely candidate for hypogonadism, a medical condition in which the sex glands produce few or no hormones.

"Generally, the lower limit of normal testosterone is around 240—if you're under that number, a doctor would consider you to be testosterone deficient and a candidate for testosterone replacement," says Dr. Saltman. "Patients that have a testosterone level between 240 and 300 fall into a gray area, since that isn't necessarily that low. However, if those patients have true clinical symptoms of testosterone deficiency—such as decreased libido, erectile dysfunction, muscle weakness, or poor exercise capacity, for example—it would be reasonable to offer them a trial of testosterone replacement."

Once a patient is diagnosed by a doctor as having low T (typically through an in-office blood test), he's checked to see if that low number is due to either a testicular problem or a pituitary-gland problem.

There are two types of testosterone deficiency. The first is primary hypogonadism, in which there is an abnormality of the testicles that prevents them from producing as much testosterone. "The other form is secondary hypogonadism, in which, for reasons we don't understand, the pituitary hormones are not secreted in large enough quantities to stimulate the testicles into producing enough testosterone," says Dr. Saltman.

Anything above 1,000 ng/dl is extremely rare. However, if you're either experiencing some form of glandular cancer or receiving the hormone through artificial means (such as testosterone-replacement therapy or illegal steroids, for example), it is possible to have a T-level that exceeds 1,000 ng/dl on a more frequent basis. Most men, however, fall in the normal—albeit dropping—range of T and can benefit from taking steps to boost T.

The Three Types of T

The average testosterone levels for most men may run between 300 and 1,000 ng/dl, but that number only represents your total testosterone. There are actually three different forms of the hormone, because once it's secreted into your bloodstream, most of your testosterone becomes bound to certain types of proteins that can make your testosterone either partially active or completely inactive.

THERE'S NO 'T' IN 'AGGRESSION'

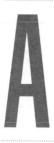

Are you worried that turning up your testosterone will turn your into a self-centered, antagonistic, antisocial brute? Despite testosterone's long-standing bad-boy reputation, there's no concrete evidence that the male hormone is the root of all aggression or violent behaviors. According to new research by Swiss neuroscientist Christoph Eisenegger, PhD, testosterone may actually cause people to act more fairly and behave more altruistically in certain situations.

The University of Zurich researcher placed more than 120 subjects in a common behavioral experiment in which two people were asked to negotiate dividing a specific amount of money. In the experiment, the first subject (the proposer) recommends how to split the cash, and the second subject (the responder) can either accept or decline the offer. If the responder accepts the proposal, the money is given to both subjects, but if the responder declines it, neither subject receives any money. Four hours before the game started, subjects were given either 0.5 milligrams of testosterone or a placebo. They were also queried about whether they believed they had been given the real testosterone or the placebo.

Dr. Eisenegger anticipated that if testosterone truly caused aggression, the T-boosted subjects would use more aggressive, egocentric, and risky strategies to present lower, unfair offers. Yet, to the researcher's surprise, subjects who were given testosterone predominantly offered better—and fairer—offers than did the people who weren't juiced up on testosterone. Even more surprising was the fact that subjects who believed they had been administered testosterone tended to act greedy and make conspicuously unfair offers. That result suggests that the mere assumption that testosterone influences aggressive behavior—not the hormone itself—may have caused the people to act more aggressively. Dr. Eisenegger believes the actual hormone's effect on behavior is dependent on the situation. Testosterone, he says, fuels the drive toward success. In situations in which cooperation is crucial to winning, as in the money game in the study, the hormone may influence fair play and cooperation to reach that goal.

"Free" (or unbound) testosterone is the hormone in its purest form, without a single molecule of protein clinging to it. In free form, testosterone is the most biologically active and able to pull off all of the jobs mentioned throughout this chapter. Unfortunately, free testosterone makes up only about 2 to 3 percent of what you actually have circulating through your body.

The second type is SHBG-bound testosterone, which is testosterone that's bound to sex-hormone-binding globulin. Produced by your liver, SHBG's job is to control the amount of free testosterone you have flowing through your body. The more SHBG you have in your system, the less free testosterone you're likely to have in your blood, going to where it's needed. On average, about 40 to 45 percent of your total testosterone is SHBG-bound and biologically inactive.

The third form is albumin-bound testosterone, which is bound to a type of protein also made by your liver that helps stabilize extra-cellular fluid volume. In short, it prevents the liquid in your blood from leaking out into your tissues. This form makes up the rest of your total testosterone level, and because this testosterone is bound to albumin, it's inactive, too. However, since the bond between testosterone and albumin is much weaker than that between SHBG and testosterone, that bond can easily be broken, turning it into active T when your body needs more free testosterone. Because it can be changed into usable testosterone, albumin-bound T is lumped in with free testosterone and designated as bioavailable testosterone.

FACTS ABOUT THE HELPFUL HORMONE

N ow that you know it's bioavailable testosterone that you're after, let's look at what active testosterone can do for you. It doesn't just guarantee that you'll build bigger muscles; this helpful hormone sports a bunch of other benefits that make it impossible to ignore. From keeping your mind sharp and protecting you from injury to appearing more attractive to the opposite sex, testosterone works behind the scenes to keep you at the top of your game—and live longer to enjoy all its perks.

T Turns Her On

A recent study at Wayne State University pitted pairs of men against each other to win the attention of an attractive female using a simple 7-minute videotaped competition. Researchers discovered that high levels of serum testosterone were positively linked with a man's dominance behaviors in competition for a mate. Those men in the study with the highest T-levels were more assertive, took more control of the conversation, and generally clicked better with females.

T May Help You Live Longer

Studies have shown that lower testosterone levels may place you at a greater risk of death. In a study, researchers at the VA Puget Sound Health Care System's Geriatric Research Education and Clinical Centers investigated mortality-risk factors in male veterans over 40 years of age by measuring testosterone levels periodically for 4 years. They found that as subjects' testosterone levels went down, their risk of death went up. In fact, researchers found that men with low testosterone had a 68 percent greater risk of death than men with normal T-levels.

Another study, performed at the University of California at San Diego, followed 800 men (ages 50 to 91) for a period of 18 years. At the start of the study, 29 percent of the men suffered from low testosterone. During the next 18 years, those with lower amounts of testosterone had a 33 percent higher risk of death than guys with high testosterone levels, and they experienced higher levels of inflammation and had a greater likelihood of developing metabolic syndrome—a mix of medical disorders that work together to increase your risk of developing coronary artery disease, stroke, and Type 2 diabetes.

MRS. T

Testosterone may be the primary male sex hormone, but it's not exclusively a man's hormone. Women also produce androgens—including testosterone, which for women is manufactured by the ovaries and the adrenal glands—but their secretions are much smaller in concentration, roughly 10 to 20 times less than are found in men.

T Toughens Up Your Ticker

It's a common belief that higher levels of testosterone have a negative effect on heart health, especially since men are twice as likely as women to meet their demise from coronary artery disease. But although large doses of testosterone found in anabolic steroids may be harmful to health, according to a 2010 study in the United Kingdom, having high testosterone isn't what makes men susceptible to heart-health issues—it's having too little T that could be the culprit.

Researchers examined 930 men with coronary disease and tracked their heart health for an average of 7 years. Beforehand, they calculated the levels of both total testosterone and bioavailable testosterone in the subjects, and found that 20 percent of the men had clinically defined testosterone deficiency. During the 7-year span, 1 in 5 of the low-testosterone subjects died, compared with only 1 in 8 subjects who had normal T-levels. The researchers say that low testosterone may contribute to obesity, elevated harmful blood fats, and insulin resistance—each of which is a risk factor for heart disease.

T Keeps Your Brain Sharp

Society loves to assume that guys with more testosterone are too obsessed with strength and sex to think about anything cerebral, but the exact opposite is true, according to Dutch researchers. In a study, Dutch scientists evaluated the cognitive performance of 400 men between the ages of 40 and 80 and noticed a direct linear relationship between T-levels and cognitive function among the men who were 70 to 80 years old. The higher their testosterone levels, the better they performed certain cognitive functions and tasks.

Lower levels of testosterone may also make you more vulnerable to suffering from Alzheimer's disease later in life, according to a 2010 University of Hong Kong study that looked at the possibility of bioavailable testosterone as a predictor of developing the disease in older men. Researchers followed 153 men over 55 years of age, 47 of whom already had some form of mild cognitive impairment or memory loss.

After 1 year, 10 of the subjects who were part of the cognitively impaired group and also had low testosterone developed probable Alzheimer's disease. It's just one of several studies that suggest that healthy testosterone levels may defend against both mild memory difficulties and Alzheimer's disease.

T Adds Agility to Your Arsenal

There's a reason wide receivers, sprinters, and gymnasts are incredibly nimble. Having plenty of testosterone in your system prevents your body from losing muscle mass and improves vision, cognition, and neuromuscular coordination, all of which can help your physical performance and decrease your odds of falling.

A 4-year study from Oregon Health & Science University, in Portland, measured the testosterone levels and physical performance of more than 2,500 men between the ages of 65 and 99. Those in the group with the lowest T-levels were shown to be 40 percent more likely to suffer a fall than the high-T-level men in the group. And if you think that getting older makes you more clumsy, it may be low T that's tripping you up. In the study, it was the youngest men in the low-T group who recorded the most slips and trips.

HOW TO TEST YOUR T

There are several ways to find out how your testosterone levels stack up.

The most inexpensive—and least reliable—is a home saliva hormone test, available through any drugstore or online for around $30 to $40. Home tests that cost more generally measure other hormones such as DHEA, progesterone, and cortisol. They're easy. All you do is spit into a tiny container, then mail it back to the laboratory for results.

The more expensive—and more reliable—option is having a lab draw your blood and measure levels of either total testosterone or free testosterone or a combination of the two. Prices range from $50 to $150. "If you're serious about being evaluated for whether or not you may have testosterone deficiency, then having it done through a physician's office is a very simple, inexpensive way to check your testosterone," advises Dr. Saltman.

Whichever method you choose, give the sample first thing in the morning, between 8 and 10. T-levels fluctuate throughout the day. "It's the highest in the morning, then it gets lower during the day, so if you check your testosterone level at 4 p.m. and it's significantly lower, that number may not mean much," says Dr. Saltman.

T Keeps Old Guys from Becoming Frail

If we're fortunate to keep on living, we will get old. That's something you have no control over. But you can do something to avoid becoming a bony whisper of your former self or at least putting it off as long as possible. How? By keeping the testosterone flowing. A new study accepted by The Endocrine Society's *Journal of Clinical Endocrinology & Metabolism* shows that maintaining high testosterone levels as you age may help you preserve muscle mass and avoid becoming frail from 65 onward. Researchers from five universities analyzed testosterone levels, body composition, and physical strength in 1,183 men age 65 or older for more than 4 years and found that men with the highest testosterone levels lost the least amount of muscle mass in their arms and legs even as they lost weight with age. Older guys who had the highest testosterone could stand up more easily from a chair than men who had lower testosterone levels. The study adds more evidence that higher testosterone levels may help older men preserve muscle and delay frailty as they age, says lead study author Erin LeBlanc, MD, of Kaiser Permanente Northwest in Portland, OR.

T Strengthens Your Bones

Most men don't even bother to worry about osteoporosis, because the disease, marked by loss of bone density, is typically considered a women's problem. But they should worry; this debilitating disease affects men, too. "There's no question that men with a testosterone deficiency have a much higher incidence of osteoporosis," says Dr. Saltman.

In one Australian study, researchers investigated the connection between T-levels and the fracture risk of older men by collecting information on the bone mineral density, lifestyle factors, and testosterone levels of more than 600 older men (aged 60 years plus). After tracking the group for an average of 6 years, researchers found that lower T-levels were associated with a higher risk of low-trauma fractures.

T Fights Depression

Maybe it's just a side effect of knowing you're all man, but banking more testosterone may impact your odds of feeling depressed. When Australian researchers performed a cross-sectional study that compared the free testosterone levels and information on the psychological and physical health of nearly 4,000 men, they found that older men with lower free T-levels (below 6 ng/dl) had three times the risk of developing depression of men with high free T-levels (10 ng/dl or above).

"With the issue of depression, it can sometimes be a difficult decision in terms of what comes first—the cart or the horse," says Dr. Saltman. "There's no question that patients who are depressed have low testosterone levels, but we're still not quite certain whether their low T-levels cause depression or if depression causes a patient's testosterone levels to drop—acting like a self-defense mechanism designed to prevent you from doing anything that you may not be able to physically or emotionally do." Either way, ramping up your T-levels may be extra insurance against fatigue, lethargy, and depression.

A HEAVY BURDEN

How the great American lifestyle affects your health, weight, energy, and erections

03

I

t's what every man strives for: the big-money job, the big house with the three-car garage, the Sub-Zero fridge stocked with delicious food, a kegerator in the media room, and enough play money to eat at fine restaurants a couple times a week. We want to have what we want instantly, do as we please, and take what we deserve. After all, that's what being a man is all about, right? Winning big.

And you are living that dream, for the most part. As nearly a billion people worldwide lack access to clean drinking water, you're worrying about which case of microbrew to buy for your tailgate party. While 2.6 billion people around the globe try to cope with lacking proper sanitation, you're busy installing a flat-screen TV next to your dual-flush commode.

But don't feel guilty for having more than the rest of the world. Count your blessings but also recognize that we are paying a price for the luxuries of the Great American Lifestyle. Our debt is unhealthy stress, excess body weight, obesity, mental-health disorders, Type 2 diabetes, and heart disease. (The number of obese Americans has nearly tripled in the past 30 years!) The pursuit of the American Dream and our easy access to such excess hits our T-levels, too. Parts of our modern lifestyle, as the study in Chapter 1 suggests, are reducing testosterone levels in American men.

A Math Test

There's an arithmetic problem you may want to solve before you continue to read this chapter. All you need is two numbers: your weight in pounds and your height in inches.

1) Take your height in inches and square it (meaning, multiply that number by itself). For example, if you're 68 inches tall, you would get 4,624 (68 times 68).

2) Divide your weight by that new number. Using the same example, if you weigh 175 pounds, you would divide 175 by 4,624, leaving you with .0378.

3) Finally, multiply that fraction by 703. Again using our example, you would multiply .0378 by 703, leaving you with 26.6 as your final answer.

What did you get from your height and weight numbers? If it's what the 175-pound guy in our example came up with or higher, you're overweight. That number is your BMI, or body mass index, which serves as a simple way to measure your body fat by comparing your weight against your height. It's not an accurate science, but it's a commonly used method to gauge where you stand—or wobble.

Having a BMI greater than or equal to 25 means you're overweight. And if your numbers push 30 and above, most doctors consider you officially obese. Either way, your body is packing an abnormal amount of fat that's most likely impairing your health.

If you have a high BMI, you're far from alone. According to the World Health Organization, 1.5 billion adults worldwide are overweight, and obesity has more than doubled since 1980. In the United States alone, more than 60 percent of adults are considered overweight or obese, but is that really a big surprise?

Swallowing three square meals a day has never been easier, thanks to the convenient and inexpensive processed fare and fast food at our disposal, most of which is packed with fat, salt, and sugar.

Thanks to technology, being wired means never even having to leave your bed to connect with work, friends, and family, removing the remote possibility that you might burn a calorie or two while traveling to see a buddy, commuting to the job site, or even taking a few steps to the window to check the weather outside. I mean, why bother—there's an app for that, right?

Keeping up with the Joneses is, in all likelihood, making you fat. And if you're staring down the barrel of a BMI that's 25 or above, then you're at a much higher risk of developing some form of life-threatening and/or life-impairing disease.

You see, all that American-made adipose tissue you have hovering around your waistline makes you a prime candidate for metabolic syndrome— which is just a fancy name for a series of risk factors that are tied to being overweight or obese. Having extra fat around your middle is one of those factors, along with high blood pressure, insulin resistance, high triglyceride levels, and lower-than-normal HDL (good) cholesterol.

If the easy American way of living has led you to have at least three of these factors, then you're already at risk of developing cardiovascular disease, musculoskeletal disorders such as osteoarthritis, cancer, and Type 2 diabetes. Adult-onset diabetes is expected to affect at least 500 million people worldwide within the next two decades—all thanks to obesity.

In 2011, the Centers for Disease Control and Prevention (CDC) reported that 26 million people in the United States—8.3 percent of the population—have diabetes, which represented a 10 percent increase over the estimated number of diabetics in 2008 (23.6 million).

It's all proof positive that America is getting heavier—you along with it—and why the life you've been leading has most likely left you with a lot less testosterone than you should have.

MORE OF 'YOU' MEANS LESS OF 'T'

 ven if you couldn't care less about how your spare tire places you in danger of disease, consider this: According to a study performed at the State University of New York at Buffalo, being obese can also dramatically decrease your testosterone levels. When researchers sought to determine the frequency of below-normal concentrations of testosterone in patients with obesity or Type 2 diabetes, they discovered that 40 percent of obese participants involved in their study had lower-than-normal testosterone—a percentage that soared to 50 percent among obese men who also had diabetes. The research concluded that as body mass index increased in men, their free testosterone decreased.

That means that the wider you are around the middle, the less testosterone you probably have shooting through your system. Letting that lazy lifestyle lower your testosterone levels means looking forward to weaker and fewer erections, a lower libido, a loss of energy, and less muscle—and that's just for starters.

Here are some other testosterone saboteurs:

Your Desk Job

Your great-grand-pop probably swung a pick axe in a coal mine or plowed a field or shouldered loads on a shipping dock. In other words, he was on his feet most of the day, using his muscles to make a buck. You probably sit at a desk in front of a computer screen. You probably don't break a sweat all day until you reach the gym.

According to a study by the Washington State Department of Health, only about 6.5 percent of American adults actually meet the minimum weekly aerobic-physical-activity guidelines from their day jobs. That means that 93.5 percent of all adults have a job that's so pathetically sedentary, it doesn't even meet the minimal amount of physical activity recommended to maintain optimal health.

And the job you're doing is probably becoming easier and easier—at least from a calorie-burning standpoint. When researchers from the Pennington Biomedical Research Center, in Baton Rouge, Louisiana, examined the level of physical activity among US occupations over the past 50 years, their hope was to find a connection between occupational physical activity (the energy expenditure you spend on the job) and the concurrent increase in body weight in the United States.

Well, the Pennington researchers found a connection, all right—and your T-levels are not going to like it. According to their data, only 20 percent of jobs today require at least moderately intense physical activity, compared with almost half of jobs in the early 1960s. Worse yet, the researchers noticed that, on average, men burn 142 fewer calories on the job today than they did 50 years ago. That works out to more than 700 calories fewer each week—or almost 37,000 annually—and since 1 pound of fat equals 3,500 excess calories, that means you could be packing on an extra 10 pounds a year more than Granddaddy did 50 years ago.

Your Seniority

As we mentioned earlier, Father Time plays a cruel trick on your manhood by slowly reducing your body's testosterone production, as well as your metabolic rate—the rate at which your body burns calories at rest. Since less energy spent equals more energy stored, that slower metabolism leads to an increase in overall body fat, which in turn further reduces testosterone levels.

Your Soap

There's a reason men were meant to have a little dirt under their fingernails: It keeps us from turning into women. You see, some soaps and personal-care products contain an additive called triclocarban (TCC), an antimicrobial ingredient that can cause health problems by interfering with your body's normal hormone action.

Other popular additives that could be attacking your testosterone levels are lavender and tea tree oil. A study performed at the National Institute of Environmental Health Sciences, in North Carolina, found that these ingredients, commonly found in shampoos, soaps, and lotions, were the culprits behind a

hormonal imbalance between estrogen and testosterone in young boys—
an imbalance that caused them to experience abnormal breast development
(otherwise known as gynecomastia).

Scientists discovered that both oils seem to have an estrogenlike effect on
human breast-cancer cells, while they also suppressed responsiveness to
male hormones. Once the subjects stopped using products with either
ingredient, the estrogenic conditions abated as well.

Your Stress Levels

Stress hormones are stress hormones, whether you're worried about being
threatened by a saber-toothed tiger or by foreclosure on your home. Either
way, your body assumes you need instant energy to either fight off what's
stressing you or run away from it as fast as possible, so it triggers the release
of cortisol and adrenaline, two hormones that can hinder many of your
body's anabolic functions, particularly testosterone production. The
problem is that tiger-attack stress is short-lived: Either you're dead or
you've made a successful escape. Bankers, the IRS, the economic downturn—
all those modern bullies are much more dogged. They last and last and last,
keeping you up nights and causing chronic anxiety all day. Long-term stress
is the worst kind.

Of the two stress hormones excreted during times of fear and challenge,
cortisol is your worst nightmare, since it's catabolic in nature (meaning that
its job is to break down larger molecules—in this case, your muscles—into
smaller units of energy). Whenever stress strikes, cortisol goes to work
converting amino acids from within your muscles into carbohydrates—
essentially tearing down your muscles to give your body extra energy that it
doesn't even need.

Cortisol also prevents your muscles from storing glycogen, and it interferes
with how effectively testosterone can bind to its receptors within muscle cells,
which essentially lowers your T-levels. But to add insult to injury, falling
T-levels give the estrogen in your system the opportunity to make a bigger
impact on your body. With less testosterone to counterbalance that extra
estrogen, your body will find it more difficult to shed body fat, and your gut will
grow. The more body fat you're packing, the less testosterone your body will
end up producing. It's a vicious cycle that sends your T into the toilet.

Your Sleep

When a guy's list of priorities becomes too much to bear, something's got to go. And usually he finds that sleep is the most easily expendable. That's bad news for testosterone and other hormones that do their best work when we are at rest.

Fewer hours of sleep generally means less deep sleep, the kind you get during non-REM stages 3 and 4 in your sleep cycle. This is the slow-brain-wave sleep that's necessary for restoring your body. Deep sleep plays a crucial role in maintaining good general health, and it's absolutely essential for repairing the damaged tissues in your body.

Human growth hormone (HGH)—the body's rejuvenating hormone—is released primarily during the deep-sleep stages. HGH is a protein that accelerates the movement of amino acids through cell membranes and boosts protein synthesis. Growth hormone's main job is to stimulate muscle repair, enzyme production, and cell replacement. It even revitalizes the immune system, which is why it's so easy to come down with a cold after you pull an all-nighter. But much worse than triggering the sniffles, lack of adequate sleep floods your body with cortisol, placing your body in a higher catabolic state that consumes muscle and stores body fat.

RAISE YOUR BMI—AND TELL T BYE-BYE

Even the slightest change in your body mass index (BMI) can have a huge effect on your testosterone production. When researchers at the New England Research Institutes performed a study to confirm that certain health and lifestyle changes could significantly lower testosterone levels in men, they found that an increase of a mere 4 to 5 points in BMI had the same impact on lowering a man's total testosterone as did 10 years of aging.

Your Environment

Thanks to plastic, you've been able to enjoy food in convenient on-the-go ways that your icebox-dependent forefathers could only dream of. But what science failed to tell you is that a chemical called bisphenol A (BPA), used to make plastic food and drink containers, has been slowly chipping away at your testosterone. BPA is even in the cans you probably have lining your pantry—a 2011 study performed by the US Food and Drug Administration detected the harmful chemical in 71 out of 78 random canned food products.

BPA has become one of the world's highest-production-volume chemicals, and because of that popularity it is now found inside more than 90 percent of the world's population. Being exposed to the chemical has been linked to a host of health issues, including thyroid hormone disruption, cardiovascular disease, and obesity. One of the reasons BPA is so harmful is that it's an endocrine disruptor that mimics your body's hormones. It's a trick that can interfere with the production of hormones like testosterone. By mimicking estrogen in your system, BPA can cause your body to store excess body fat, and the more fat you have, the more frequently that fat takes whatever

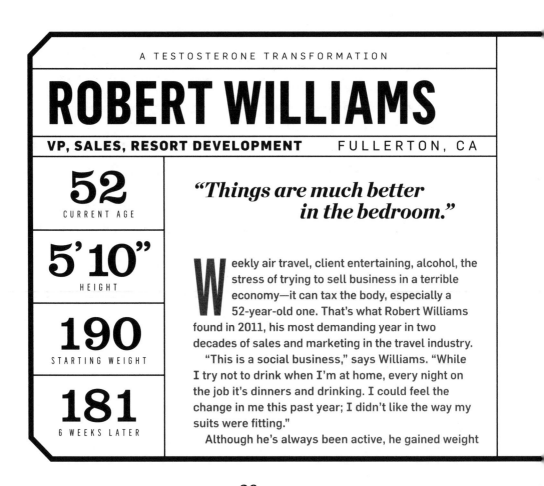

A TESTOSTERONE TRANSFORMATION

ROBERT WILLIAMS

VP, SALES, RESORT DEVELOPMENT   FULLERTON, CA

52
CURRENT AGE

5'10"
HEIGHT

190
STARTING WEIGHT

181
6 WEEKS LATER

"Things are much better in the bedroom."

Weekly air travel, client entertaining, alcohol, the stress of trying to sell business in a terrible economy—it can tax the body, especially a 52-year-old one. That's what Robert Williams found in 2011, his most demanding year in two decades of sales and marketing in the travel industry.

"This is a social business," says Williams. "While I try not to drink when I'm at home, every night on the job it's dinners and drinking. I could feel the change in me this past year; I didn't like the way my suits were fitting."

Although he's always been active, he gained weight

testosterone you have floating in your system and converts it into estrogen.

But BPA isn't the only endocrine-disrupting chemical. Other compounds interfere with the function of your endocrine system, including certain insecticides (like carbaryl and chlorpyrifos, found in tick-and-flea powder and lawn treatments), fungicides, and other industrial chemicals (known as phthalates) that are used to make plastics more pliable.

That's right: If your testosterone is low, you might not have to look any further for the culprit than your old garden hose, your Bichon Frise, the shiny dashboard of your car, your water bottle, or even her vibrator. When it comes to natural and man-made substances ready to cause damage to your endocrine system and confuse your T-levels, the good life has your testicles surrounded.

in recent months. He felt more aches and pains and wasn't sleeping well. "I was tired and kind of blasé in the bedroom. I never had my testosterone level checked, but I knew something was different."

Williams was determined to turn things around, so he started looking for a fitness program. "I wanted to think out of the box, then this Testosterone Transformation workout came a long. I thought, "Wow, this is heavy duty.' I had never done this kind of exercise. I loved its intensity."

RESULTS: After 6 weeks on the program, Williams dropped 9 pounds, built solid muscle, and improved his flexibility. His waist size shrunk from 37 to 33 as the pounds melted away.

His wife, was amazed by how quickly he trimmed his belly. "Things are much better in the bedroom," Williams says. "And that's a big deal. I have greater interest and energy for sex and more frequent erections."

But the most significant change, Williams admits, is that he has reduced his alcohol consumption by more than 60 percent. "The workouts are brutal. No way could I pull them off if I was drinking like I used to. So the program has had a considerable impact on every aspect of my health, my sex life, and my strength."

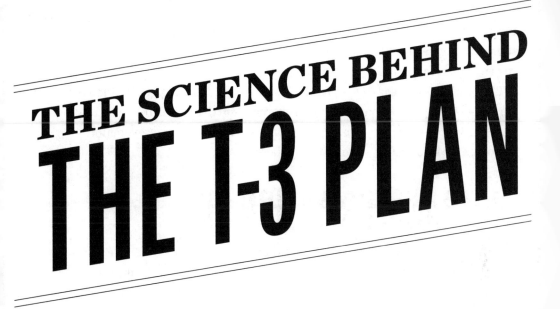

THE SCIENCE BEHIND THE T-3 PLAN

An introduction to the program that will change your life

CHAPTER

04

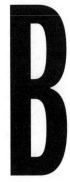

y now, two things should be abundantly clear to you: Testosterone is crucial to being the best man you can be and living a long, fruitful, and happy life. You've also learned that while your T-levels may fluctuate greatly throughout the day, they certainly decline throughout the years beyond age 30. But you can do something about that. It just takes the right plan to help your body fight back.

The foundation of the *Men's Health* Testosterone Transformation Plan is a three-tiered approach that focuses on exercise, nutrition, and lifestyle. It will help you to lose body fat quickly, gain more muscle, and release even more testosterone into your system than ever before.

T1: TRANSFORMATION DIET

O ne of the most effective ways to increase testosterone is through diet, because nutrients and hormones (like testosterone) work hand in hand in regulating the process that repairs muscle tissue broken down during resistance training. As you know, this muscle-protein breakdown/buildup process is the mechanism by which your muscle and strength grow. But it doesn't work optimally if your diet doesn't supply the correct building blocks.

Unfortunately, if you've been following the traditional advice for losing weight—cut calories, reduce fat in your diet, and watch your intake of red meat and eggs—you are going to miss out on those critical nutrients that foster "anabolism," or muscle buildup. The advice you've heard from doctors, the popular media, and nagging loved ones for years is simply wrong. If you've been following that advice, it may be why you're not building the kind of muscle you're after. What the "experts" neglected to tell you is that all of those "healthy" eating tips are three of the fastest ways to drop your testosterone levels from a drenching to a drip.

The key nutrient known to influence testosterone production most dramatically is fat. In fact, studies show that limiting fat to 10 percent or less of your total calories can significantly reduce your testosterone levels. The total number of calories consumed has a direct relationship to testosterone levels, too. Studies in which men were put on low-calorie diets (about 1,800 calories per day) while doing exhaustive exercise found that testosterone had decreased 40 to 50 percent after just 5 days. And another study of 1,522 men aged 40 to 70 found that men following low-protein diets had decreased testosterone and lower sex drives.

That's why eating to lose body fat while simultaneously eating to gain testosterone is a tricky road to travel. You need enough calories, fat, and protein for optimum testosterone without taking in an excess of calories that can be stored as fat. Fortunately, the Testosterone Transformation Diet will show you how to eat the right combination of foods—at the right times of the day—to lose belly fat, curb production of the stress hormone cortisol, and boost testosterone secretion for maximum muscle growth.

The best part is that our nutrition program looks nothing like the highly restrictive, super-detailed eating plans that you may be used to, diets that are difficult to stick with. The T-Transformation Diet is different because, well, it's not a traditional diet at all. The classic dietary commandments—restricting calories, cutting fat, eating less red meat and eggs and a lot more fiber—are a recipe for lowering T-levels. For robust T-levels, this diet will require you to eat more food (to fuel all the hard exercise you'll be doing), get your fill of quality protein like red meat and fish, and keep your consumption of calories from fat—preferably heart-healthy monounsaturates and omega-3s—above 30 percent. In short, you'll be eating many of the foods you already love. I don't expect to hear any complaints about the food on this program.

T2: TRANSFORMATION WORKOUT

L osing the belly fat responsible for inflating your estrogen levels and crushing your T-levels may seem easy enough, especially if you assume that the best solution is a regular exercise regime. But there's a big catch to that belief. Although regular exercise can help you blast off body fat, if it's done incorrectly—which is what most men are already guilty of—then you can actually bring your T-levels to a screeching halt. For example, one study found that intense long-distance running can dramatically lower testosterone.

How you train, how often you train, and how quickly you lose body fat can all play an important part in deciding how much testosterone your body either makes or misses. Even choosing the number of times to lift a weight has a bearing on which hormones your body chooses to ooze.

A 2011 study performed at the Laboratory for Clinical and Experimental Research in Vascular Biology at the State University of Rio de Janeiro, Brazil, looked at the effect of resistance-training volume on the hormonal responses—particularly testosterone, growth hormone, cortisol, and the testosterone/cortisol ratio—in men. Their subjects were asked to perform two identical workouts one week apart using the same exercises—barbell bench presses, leg presses, lat pulldowns, leg curls, shoulder abductions, and leg extensions. The only difference in the workouts was the volume. For the first workout, subjects performed 3 sets of each exercise using 80 percent of their 6-rep maximum (the greatest amount of weight they could lift 6 times). For the second workout, subjects performed 3 sets of each exercise using 80 percent of their 12-rep maximum. The researchers found that testosterone and HGH (human growth hormone) levels significantly increased in men performing either workout. However, the men experienced significantly higher levels of cortisol, as well as a lower testosterone/cortisol ratio, when performing the higher-rep sets—confirming that volume is an important factor when it comes to your body's hormonal response to resistance training.

Even pushing yourself too hard in an attempt to burn calories and blast away fat can block your body from getting its fill of testosterone. Overtraining does more than tax your immune system and increase your risk of becoming too sick to exercise—it can also raise your body's concentration of catabolic (breaking-down) hormones, particularly cortisol, and lower its levels of muscle-building anabolic hormones.

Resistance training done the right way is the key to more T. Weight lifting sets the stage for testosterone to act as a muscle builder—almost as if you were injecting yourself with a natural, healthy dose of steroids, William Kraemer, PhD, a kinesiology researcher at the University of Connecticut's Human Performance Laboratory, told *Men's Health*.

The T-Transformation Workout factors in all of the exercise issues that can send your body into shutdown mode and instead flips all the switches that ensure your body reacts to every workout the way you want it to—with a big burst of T!

For example, our workout discourages aerobic exercise because it can actually lower testosterone. For maximum T production, our formula relies on compound weight-lifting exercises, multijoint lifts that stimulate the most muscle tissue, using heavy weights, and limiting rest between sets.

The workouts in this book also affect other key anabolic hormones—growth hormone, in particular. Growth hormone helps your body synthesize protein so you'll build more muscle faster. It is also critical in decreasing your body's use of glucose and encouraging the breakdown of unwanted body fat, so you have less blubber covering up your newly built muscles. Short rest periods during weight lifting are particularly effective at increasing growth-hormone concentrations in muscle, according to a recent study in the *Journal of Strength and Conditioning Research*.

T3: TRANSFORMATION LIFESTYLE

ou can master everything possible when it comes to your diet-and-exercise regime, but if you think those are the only two tools of the trade that, when combined, will bring you all the T you need, then life has a few surprises for you. With so many environmental pitfalls waiting out there, each ready to take its turn at hammering down your T-levels, you need a game plan that can walk you through all of the everyday hazards that can collectively have a debilitating effect on how much testosterone your body is able to produce.

Just like the T-Transformation Diet, the T-Transformation Lifestyle isn't as difficult as the title may imply.

Instead, you'll follow a simple series of do's and don'ts throughout the day, from getting the right amount of sleep to dodging certain products that may be elevating the estrogen in your bloodstream. The more do's you can achieve in your daily routine—and the more don'ts you can avoid—the higher you can expect to see your T-levels rise.

When all three steps of the T-Transformation Plan are combined, they add up to a 12-week routine that does more than blast off your belly fat and pack on premium muscle. It's a system that will push your T-levels through the ceiling, offering you more energy and a stronger sex drive, while lowering your risk of metabolic syndrome, diabetes, heart disease, and erectile dysfunction.

Now that you know the steps, it's time to take the first one in Chapter 5.

PROTEIN

The building block of muscle

CHAPTER

05

A

fter oxygen, sand is the most abundant element on Earth. It's everywhere, in every crack and crevice. It even gets into your own cracks and crevices after a day at the beach.

Well, you can think of protein the same way. After water, protein is the most common substance in your body. It makes up about one-fifth of your muscles (the rest being primarily water), but that's only a small part of your protein connection. "You find a little bit of it in every cell of your body, including in your organs, hair, nails, and skin," says Tara Gidus, RD, CSSD, LD/N, team nutritionist for the Orlando Magic.

Most nutritionists, physiologists, and doctors refer to protein as "the building block of life," because without this important macronutrient your body wouldn't be able to build any part of itself at all.

You probably haven't thought of protein this way before, but it's rather crucial to your existence. Here are some other reasons why it plays a prominent role in the Testosterone Transformation Diet, according to Gidus:

▶ Protein constructs and repairs body tissues, and not just the muscular kind but cartilage, bones, organs, and connective tissue.

▶ Protein produces the enzymes that digest food.

▶ Protein is found in antibodies that keep you healthy by resisting diseases.

▶ Protein regulates body processes such as water balancing, oxygen and energy transportation, and making muscles contract.

▶ Protein is involved in dozens of other areas that can affect how your body functions, how it looks, and how much testosterone it's able to produce.

Protein Builds Muscle without Making You Fat

Eat too many calories and one thing's for certain: Your body will assume that anything extra in your tank is something you want to store for later. That reaction can cause your body to pack on unwanted fat, but that's not as easy to do when you eat protein.

The reason many men get fat from eating too many carbs is simple—as in simple sugars. Most carb-rich foods are packed with simple sugars that raise your body's blood-glucose levels. "Your body's natural response to all that excess sugar is to release excess insulin, which causes your body to quickly metabolize all those extra calories and store them as fat," says Gidus.

Protein doesn't evoke the same waist-inflating insulin jolt because it lacks the simple sugars that carbohydrates have. Its job is to accelerate muscle growth by rebuilding stressed muscles after vigorous exercise.

Protein Fills You Up

Protein makes your stomach feel full quicker, and research has shown that it takes about 2 hours longer than carbohydrates to digest, so you won't get hungry again as soon.

"One reason many men tend to overeat and store more body fat is because they aren't eating the right balance of macronutrients," says Gidus. "Carbohydrates are converted, digested, and utilized at a much faster pace than protein, which is why you may still feel hungry after eating a carb-loaded meal. Fat takes the longest to digest, which is why you may eat too much of a fat-rich food before finally feeling full."

Protein falls right in the middle—it takes much longer than carbs to digest and it's more readily converted into energy than fat is. Getting enough protein ensures that you'll have enough of each macronutrient so that you always have a steady stream of energy available to your body. By regulating blood-sugar levels, protein helps prevent the wild swings that cause you to binge.

Protein Puts Up a Metabolic Fight

Digesting your food requires a certain amount of energy, and protein requires more than carbs do to process. In a study performed at the Department of Nutrition at Arizona State University East, researchers discovered that eating a high-protein diet caused subjects' bodies to burn twice as many calories—or about an extra 30 calories burned per meal. The more calories you can burn off without expending any extra effort, the less body fat you'll be saddled with to hamper your production of testosterone.

OPTIMUM PROTEIN

ith so much going for protein, you might start contemplating raising cattle in your backyard. But you can consume too much of a good thing—there's only so much protein your body can process.

"Once your body has enough for what it needs to rebuild muscle, it breaks down protein and stores it as body fat," says Gidus.

Generally, for healthy people, following a high-protein diet is fairly safe in the short term. But eating too much protein can potentially exacerbate liver and kidney problems for anyone who may already have trouble eliminating the waste products of protein metabolism. Whenever your body breaks down protein into glucose, it needs to remove both nitrogen and ammonia from the molecule (the ammonia being a by-product of the process). "Both of those actions require fluid," says Gidus, "which is why it's important to remain hydrated when eating a high-protein diet."

So what's the best formula for safe and effective protein eating? The Dietary Reference Intake (DRI) recommendation for daily protein for men is 0.8 grams for every kilogram (2.2 pounds) of body weight—or 0.36 grams per pound. However, this is a minimum amount of protein. The exercises in this book are challenging and designed to maximize muscle production, so you're going to need more protein than the average couch potato. Research shows that athletes—particularly those who are training to build more muscle—require much more protein. "Athletes who strength-train need 1.6 to 1.7 grams per kilogram of body weight, which is twice as much as the DRI for protein," says Gidus. That's roughly 0.72 to 0.77 grams per pound.

If you have money to burn, and feel like doubling or tripling that number, then know this: You'd be wasting your time. "Your body can't process more than one gram of protein per pound of body weight each day," Gidus says. That means that if you weigh 190 pounds, then between 136 and 146 grams of protein is optimum. That's about 584 calories' worth of protein, since every gram of protein contains 4 calories. Anything over 190 grams doesn't help.

BEST SOURCES OF PROTEIN

T o you, sitting down to a steak dinner may be an occasion, but to your muscles it's more of an equation.

You see, protein is actually made up of a series of smaller particles called amino acids. Your body needs exactly 20 different types of amino acids in order to pull off all of the things mentioned in this chapter, but your body is able to produce only 11 of them. It can't manufacturer the other nine, which are histidine, isoleucine, leucine, lysine, methionine, phenylalanine, threonine, trypto-phan, and valine. These nine are called essential amino acids, because it's essential for good health that you get them from your food.

Proteins, however, are not all created equal. Some sources contain fewer amino acids, and some proteins don't contain all of the essential nine. Those that do contain all nine—meats, poultry, fish, eggs, soy, tofu, and most protein powders—earn the distinction of being called complete proteins. Those are the proteins you want to set your sights on, the ones that give you the biggest boost for T-produc-tion and muscle growth.

Among the complete proteins, beef is your T-level's best choice. Loaded with protein, beef also provides other nutrients that are pro-anabolic. First, every cut has a certain amount of saturated fats and cholesterol, which, as we'll explain in the next chapter, are key to raising your T-levels. Beef also contains ample amounts of body-boosting nutrients such as iron and B-12, as well as creatine, zinc, and magnesium. And grass-fed beef also contains conjugated linoleic acid (CLA), which studies have shown helps reduce belly fat and build lean muscle.

THE LATEST ON SOY

S oy protein—derived from defatted soybean meal—is a complete protein, like beef and eggs, meaning it contains the nine essential amino acids humans need. That would make it a good T-booster as well. But soy and soy products like tofu have for many years been thought to send T-levels spiraling downward. The reason: Soy contains isoflavones, a class of organic chemicals that can act like estrogen in your body. However, recent research has shown that soy has no effect on testosterone. A 2010 study performed at St. Catherine University, in St. Paul, Minnesota, measured testosterone levels in a group of men who were given soy foods to eat. The researchers were trying to determine whether ingesting soy protein or isoflavones would produce estrogen-like effects. The researchers discovered that soy foods had no impact on testosterone at all. "Feel free to eat soy-based protein in powder and tofu to your heart's content," says Gidus. "In fact, your heart may thank you for it, since the isoflavones found in soy also have been shown to help prevent cardio-vascular disease, as well as certain types of cancer, including colorectal and prostate cancer."

Poultry shares top billing among the protein elite, especially because there's a healthy limit when it comes to how much saturated fat and cholesterol you should eat. Although darker cuts of poultry have amounts of cholesterol similar to red meat's, lean poultry has less cholesterol—as well as less saturated fat. To hit your protein requirements, eat skinless white-meat poultry (in addition to lean red meat) to avoid exceeding the heart-healthy guidelines for fat and cholesterol.

Eating fish also helps you reach your daily quota of protein (without breaking the fat bank) by providing all nine essential amino acids and much lower amounts of saturated fat. Bonus: Cold-water fish like salmon and tuna contain an abundance of heart-healthy omega-3 fatty acids (specifically DHA and EPA) so you get your good fats while eating your healthy protein. And some fish also provide a muscle-boosting shot of the compound creatine. Herring offers the most creatine per pound that you can get in any food source (3 to 4 grams per pound, while beef and pork contain 2 grams per pound).

Dairy products (milk, cheese, and yogurt) and eggs each have their place in the complete-protein department as well—with some being more helpful to your T-levels than others. For example, whole eggs deliver not only plenty of protein but also cholesterol, which is essential for making testosterone. It's now widely held that eating an egg or two daily is no longer considered the heart-disease no-no it once was. In fact, a recent study in the *Journal of Nutrition* found that eating eggs increases the beneficial HDL cholesterol without affecting LDL.

Finally, there's powdered protein. Various brands derive their protein from different sources, such as dairy products, soy, and eggs. Powdered protein supplements are so popular because of convenience: They require no cooking or refrigeration. It's instant protein—just mix with milk, water, or juice.

There are two basic types of powered proteins—whey and casein—and each acts a bit differently in your body. Whey protein (which comes from milk) contains the highest level of branched-chain amino acids (see why BCAAs matter in Chapter 16) and is one of the fastest-digesting proteins you can eat. Because it's so quickly absorbed, whey protein is an excellent choice post-workout to jump-start muscle repair. A whey smoothie is also a terrific drink for first thing in the morning, to protect your muscles from catabolic damage. When your body is energy-deprived after a long night's sleep, it can tap your muscles as an energy source. You don't want that to happen, so make a whey smoothie part of your wake-up routine.

Casein powdered protein is also derived from milk, but it is digested by your body at a much slower pace than whey and other forms of powdered protein. It can take up to 7 hours for your body to fully process casein protein. There are advantages to this drawn-out process. For one, the longer it takes to digest, the more calories your body naturally burns doing so, which gives you an extra fat-loss benefit. Second, because casein protein is absorbed slowly, your muscles receive a steady stream of amino acids for hours at a time. That's why casein is the preferred choice for right before bedtime. It provides a constant flow of amino acids throughout the night, when your body is hard at work repairing muscles.

Incomplete Protein Sources

With the exception of soy, hemp, and quinoa (a tasty high-protein grain), most plants do not contain all of the essential amino acids. Grains, legumes (beans), nuts, seeds, and certain vegetables all contain some amount of protein but lack one or more of the essential amino acids, so they are referred to as incomplete proteins.

So where does that leave your muscles and your T-levels, especially if you're a vegetarian and prefer to rely on these types of foods for protein instead of meats, dairy products, and eggs? By eating the right two incomplete protein sources—either within the same meal or during the course of the day—your body can get all nine essential amino acids that it needs.

For example, chickpeas and sesame seeds are both incomplete protein sources, but mix them up in hummus and you create a complete protein that can be just as effective at providing all nine essential amino acids as anything you'll get from a cow, chicken, fish, or other living, breathing creature. The best thing about combining incomplete proteins is that you don't have to be a genius to do it. It's as simple as mixing either:

▶ a grain and a legume (such as rice and beans)

▶ a legume and nuts or seeds (such as hummus or trail mix)

▶ some nuts or seeds and a grain

WHY TEAMING UP IS BETTER FOR YOUR T-LEVELS

Mixing your protein sources isn't just for vegetarians—it's a smart thing to do even if you're planning to stick to eating complete sources of protein. A lot of guys make the mistake of getting in a rut with the proteins they turn to. If they like chicken, they eat nothing but chicken. If they like eggs and beef, they stick to that. It can become boring fast.

Here's what you need to know: Even if a food contains all nine essential

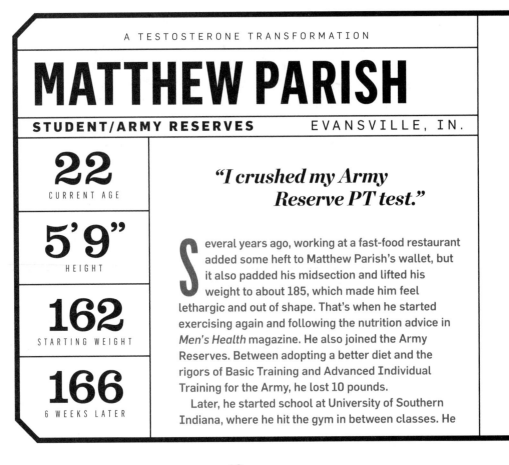

A TESTOSTERONE TRANSFORMATION

MATTHEW PARISH

STUDENT/ARMY RESERVES   EVANSVILLE, IN.

22
CURRENT AGE

5'9"
HEIGHT

162
STARTING WEIGHT

166
6 WEEKS LATER

"I crushed my Army Reserve PT test."

Several years ago, working at a fast-food restaurant added some heft to Matthew Parish's wallet, but it also padded his midsection and lifted his weight to about 185, which made him feel lethargic and out of shape. That's when he started exercising again and following the nutrition advice in *Men's Health* magazine. He also joined the Army Reserves. Between adopting a better diet and the rigors of Basic Training and Advanced Individual Training for the Army, he lost 10 pounds.

Later, he started school at University of Southern Indiana, where he hit the gym in between classes. He

amino acids, it doesn't mean it contains an equal amount of all nine. That's because every protein source is different when it comes to how much of each amino acid it has within it.

For example, legumes have less of the amino acids tryptophan, methionine, and cystine, even though they are richer in the amino acids lysine and isoleucine. Alternately, most seeds and nuts are packed with tryptophan, methionine, and cystine. Complete protein sources are just as diverse, with some containing more of one amino acid and less of another.

That's why Gidus recommends getting a variety of proteins in your diet. "You'll improve your odds of getting enough of each essential amino acid by eating different protein foods each day," she says. Variety is not only the spice of life; it's also what can lead to more muscle.

trimmed down to 162 lean pounds, but then he wanted to pack on muscle.

"I was looking for something to help me get bigger and stronger," says Parish. "I was having trouble increasing my bench press." Parish learned about the Testosterone Transformation test panel and eagerly signed up.

"This program is intense," he says. "For the first couple of weeks, the day after the upper body workouts, I could hardly move."

The soreness meant the workouts were working. "You only get out of it what you put into it," he says. By the fourth week, Parish saw the veins starting to pop on his arms, and his chest and legs were noticeably bigger.

The meal plan was easy for him because he had already trimmed his carbohydrate consumption. He has a whey protein shake for breakfast and as a post-workout refueling; turkey sandwich lunches; and he snacks constantly on nuts.

RESULTS: The program, he says, helps him sleep great, 7 to 8 hours a night, and to wake up fresh. "I have a lot more energy," he says. "This workout has a great variety of exercises. And I love the rest intervals in between because it keeps my heart rate up just enough without exhausting my muscles too fast."

After 6 weeks, Parish added about 4 pounds of muscle to his frame. And the boost in strength impressed his staff sergeant during his recent physical training test, where he aced the pushup and sit-up tests. "This program definitely helped me add muscle and strength."

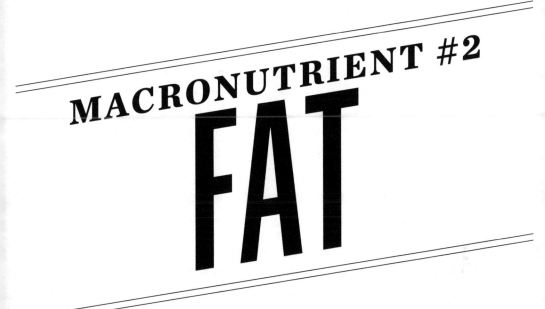

MACRONUTRIENT #2
FAT

MACRONUTRIENT #2

The truth about this much misunderstood nutrient

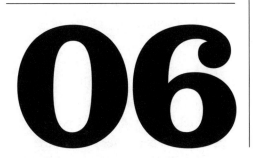

06

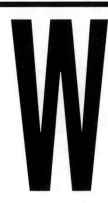

Welcome to your advanced course on fat.

Forget everything from Fat 101, where you learned that eating fat makes you fat.

That's just a big fat lie. This chapter will help you to rethink your nutrition from the ground up. It'll challenge the conventional wisdom you've been taught up until now, and some of what I tell you may sound counterintuitive. Like this: If you want to build muscle, you need to eat fat. If you've been adhering to the traditional school of thought about cutting fat from your diet in order to trim down and muscle up, you could be lowering your testosterone levels and making it harder to gain strength and mass.

THE FOUR FATS

D ietary fat is one of the three macronutrients—along with protein and carbohydrates—that your body uses for energy. And it suffers from the world's worst case of bad PR. Here's why: The tasty fat that rims your rib-eye shares the same three-letter F-word with the loathsome fat that tests the strength of your button-fly jeans. It even jiggles the same way. Dietary fat contains about 9 calories, nearly double the amount found in the other macronutrients. The federal government had a hand in creating the fat phobia, too, by advising strict limits on fat intake through its dietary guidelines. Until recently, no one had ever heard of "healthy fats." All of this perpetuated the "less fat is better" mentality.

But body fat—the tissue produced by your body—is not the same as dietary fat. And many studies have shown that cutting way back on dietary fat doesn't necessarily reduce body fat or even lower heart-disease risk. Nutrition scientists have proven that dietary fat is essential for maintaining good health. While there's still a negative stigma attached to fat, people are starting to better understand its role in the body and the fact that the four types of dietary fat are very different, too. Here's a refresher:

MONOUNSATURATED FATS. Found in an assortment of foods and oils, monounsaturated fats typically stay liquid at room temperature but tend to turn solid when chilled. Monounsaturated fats, nicknamed MUFAs, wear the "healthy fat" badge primarily because they can positively impact your heart health. Research has shown that eating foods rich in MUFAs can help bring

down blood levels of low-density lipoprotein (LDL), the so-called bad cholesterol, and reduce your risk of developing heart disease. MUFAs also might ease arthritis, protect against diabetes by stabilizing blood sugar, and ward off certain cancers. Plus, it's rich in vitamin E—an important antioxidant that most men don't get enough of, mainly because it's commonly found in fatty foods they may avoid. Studies have even shown that one particular MUFA, olive oil, prevents muscle wasting and weakness by lowering levels of a cellular protein that breaks down muscle.

Top sources of monounsaturated fat: avocados, canola oil, nuts (almonds, cashews, hazelnuts, pecans, etc.), olives and olive oil, peanut butter and peanut oil, sesame oil, sunflower oil, and even dark chocolate.

POLYUNSATURATED FATS. Known as—you guessed it—PUFAs, these plant-based oils are typically liquid both at room temperature and when chilled. PUFAs also improve blood cholesterol levels and decrease heart disease risk. They are rich in two essential fatty acids that your body can't produce on its own that are very important to your health: omega-3 and omega-6 fatty acids.

Commonly found in fish, seafood, some plants, and certain nut oils, these fatty acids have been shown to have an effect on many different areas of the body, including reducing inflammation in your joints, improving your skin's complexion, and even lowering your risk of arthritis and cancer.

Of the two, omega-3 fatty acids are the most important and the hardest to get. (The typical American diet is very rich in omega-6s.) Omega-3s (found in high concentrations in fish oil) are believed to strengthen your immune system and boost certain brain functions—such as memory and performance—by making your neurons more pliable. Even a slight deficiency in them has been shown to raise your risk of developing certain mental disorders, including attention-deficit disorder (ADD), dyslexia, depression, and schizophrenia.

Top sources of polyunsaturated fat: corn oil, cold-water fatty fish (herring, mackerel, salmon, sardines, tuna, trout, etc.), flaxseed, pumpkin seeds, safflower oil, sesame seeds, soybean oil, soy milk, sunflower seeds, tofu, and walnuts. Because fish can be a hassle to prepare (and some fish contain dangerous levels of mercury), consider taking daily capsules of purified fish oil to reap the benefits of omega-3s easily. The American Heart Association suggests 1,000 milligrams for patients with heart disease. Many doctors recommend at least that much to their patients without heart disease. Look for fish oil that contains the essential fatty acids EPA and DHA.

SATURATED FATS.
These fats, which mostly come from animal sources such as red meat, poultry, and dairy products, get their name from their chemical design. Unlike MUFAs and PUFAs, which have at least one double bond within their fatty-acid chains, this dietary fat has none. Instead, its chain of carbon atoms is virtually saturated with hydrogen atoms, which gives them the ability to stay solid at room temperature. Think of a stick of butter or the white waxy fat on a T-bone steak.

Saturated fat has been linked to increases in LDL cholesterol and elevated risk of cardiovascular disease. Some scientists believe it might also increase risk of developing Type 2 diabetes. Limiting the overall amount of saturated fat you eat is still a healthy practice, but not if you are replacing it with blood-sugar-raising carbohydrates. When your body releases the hormone insulin to deal with an influx of blood sugar, it also signals your liver to convert excess blood sugar into triglycerides, or fat. Remember, dietary fat, even the saturated variety, is important to good health and essential for testosterone production. And recent research suggests that the forbidden fat may actually do your heart and arteries a favor. Consider this: Some of the saturated fat in beef contains palmitic and lauric acids, both of which are known to raise total cholesterol. But research shows that while they do boost LDL (bad) cholesterol, they increase the HDL cholesterol to an even greater degree. HDL, high-density lipoprotein, is called the good cholesterol because it removes the plaque that LDL lays down on artery walls. So increasing both types of cholesterol actually reduces the proportion of bad cholesterol and lowers your risk of heart disease. What's more, nearly half of the fat found in beef is a monounsaturated fat called oleic acid, the same heart-healthy good stuff found in olive oil and avocados.

Top sources of saturated fat: beef, chicken with the skin on, pork, lamb, butter, cheese, coconut oil, egg yolks, palm oil, and whole-fat dairy products.

TRANS FATS.
Trans fats are among the worst food additives you can swallow, because they drive up LDL cholesterol while lowering the good HDL

cholesterol. That one-two punch can push your cholesterol profile into dangerous territory, boosting your risk of stroke, heart attack, and diabetes. Trans fats don't stop there. They also elevate triglycerides, a blood fat that contributes to atherosclerosis, a thickening of artery walls. These dangerous fats damage the cells lining blood vessels, too, triggering inflammation, which can cause blockages. Although tiny amounts of trans fats occur naturally in some meat and dairy products, the bulk of trans fats are found in processed foods. Trans fats are artificially made by taking unsaturated vegetable oil and adding hydrogen atoms into it, which keeps the oil from going rancid. For decades, trans fats have been a popular additive in foods, especially baked goods, to extend their shelf life.

Avoid these top sources of trans fat: candy bars, commercially prepared baked goods (cakes, cookies, doughnuts, muffins, and even pizza dough), margarine in stick form, most fried foods (such as french fries and onion rings), packaged snacks (such as potato chips, crackers, and microwavable popcorn), and vegetable shortening, to name a few. Look for the words "partially hydrogenated" in the ingredient list.

HOW FAT HELPS YOU LOSE WEIGHT

T here are three specific ways in which dietary fat can help you lose weight and trim your belly, maximize your muscle, and keep you swimming in testosterone.

Fat Satisfies

Luscious fat fills you up and keeps you from overeating carbohydrates. Fat is a slow-burning fuel source that—when mixed with the right balance of carbohydrates and proteins—can keep you feeling satiated for a longer period of time. Here's an example of a study that illustrates the weight-loss benefit of fatty foods: At Saint Louis University, in St. Louis, nutrition researchers fed two groups of people different types of breakfasts—one group ate eggs, the other ate bagels. Even though both breakfasts contained the same number of calories, the egg eaters consumed 264 fewer calories on average for the entire day. The fat and protein in the eggs satisfied their hunger longer.

The fuller you feel all day, the less likely you'll be to succumb to junk-food cravings—junk food that's typically high in blood-sugar-boosting carbs and, yes, those terrible trans fats.

Fat Moves Fat Away from Your Belly

The second way fat works behind the scenes is by preventing your body from storing body fat around your middle, next to your vital organs, where it can do the most damage. One now famous study, performed at the Lipids and Atherosclerosis Research Unit at the Reina Sofía University Hospital, in Córdoba, Spain, examined the effects of different types of diets on their patients to determine where body fat typically is distributed. The researchers found that subjects fed the high-carb diet had an increase in belly fat, while those on the MUFA-rich diet actually lost belly fat.

Fat Is a Building Block of Testosterone

As men, we want it all, don't we? We long to have the perfect package of rock-hard muscle strapped like armor on a fat-free physique. But as guys struggle to create that kind of body, most typically make nutritional mistakes that keep them from achieving their goals. They truly think that eating fat will only obscure their view of whatever muscle they're succeeding in packing on. But in reality, not eating enough fat out of fear of looking pudgy is what prevents most guys from building as much lean muscle as they can.

Fat is so instrumental in your T-levels that it's the reason you're reading a chapter about it before we even touch upon carbohydrates. We're not talking about its key role in preventing you from having a few rolls around your waist; we're referring to the fact that eating enough dietary fat is crucial for manufacturing testosterone. A Penn State University study of young adults found that those who consumed diets composed of 40 percent fat had significantly higher levels of testosterone than those with diets containing only 20 percent fat. Other studies show that diets with 30 percent fat will increase testosterone secretion. So the Testosterone Transformation nutrition plan will be asking you to make a paradigm shift—to start thinking of fat as your friend. We'll show you healthy ways to eat enough fat to keep you satisfied and boost your T.

HOW MUCH FAT (and what kind) TO EAT

bout 35 percent of the calories you will eat each day on the Testosterone Transformation Diet will come from fat, and 5 to 10 percent of that total should be saturated fats. That's right, saturated, one of the dreaded "bad" fats. To fill in the balance of your total fat calories each day, you'll be able to eat plenty of heart-healthy MUFAs, the monounsaturated fats. But here's the kicker: Stay away from eating PUFAs as much as you possibly can.

We know what you're thinking: Stay away from a fat known to be healthy? Yes. It might not make sense at first, but if your goal is to raise your testosterone levels naturally, you must limit PUFAs. A number of research studies, including one at Japan's Gifu University School of Medicine's Department of Public Health that investigated the relationships of different types of fat and hormones, show that eating polyunsaturated fats lowers testosterone levels.

So what's the benefit of making a certain percentage of your total fat intake saturated fats? For the cholesterol that's inside it—the same cholesterol that your body converts into the very substance you're seeking: testosterone. Most foods that contain saturated fat also contain cholesterol. Getting a certain amount through specific foods—particularly meat and egg yolks—can ensure you have enough on hand to convert into extra testosterone.

If the thought of having more cholesterol in your system sounds scary, don't worry. A recent study out of Texas A&M University examined 52 adults who were in good health but were not participating in any form of training program. Their research showed that, after putting subjects through fairly vigorous workouts, the more LDL cholesterol they had in their blood, the better they were able to build muscle mass through resistance training.

As I mentioned before, dietary cholesterol from saturated fats will raise your LDL cholesterol level, but it's all about balance. Certain saturated fats also boost the good HDL that removes LDL buildup on artery walls to actually reduce heart disease risk.

By following the Testosterone Transformation program, you'll lose body fat, add MUFAs and some saturated fats to your diet, cut out trans fats, and eat healthy carbohydrates—all of which will help to bring a healthy balance to your body and prime it for big muscle growth.

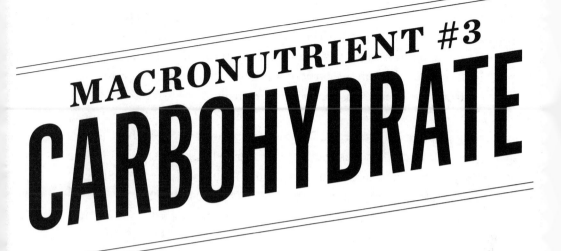

MACRONUTRIENT #3

CARBOHYDRATE

You need carbohydrates for energy, but not all are created equal

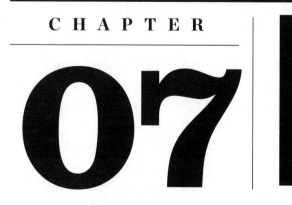

CHAPTER

07

L et's start with a silly question: Can you see yourself eating 10 slices of bread at one sitting? Okay, maybe some of you can, but most reasonable people would consider that major carb overload. Now ask yourself this:

Can you see yourself eating a common American drive-through feast—a Burger King Triple Whopper with cheese, fries, and a king-size Coke?

Yes? If you're really hungry, yes? Well, that combo meal is the equivalent of roughly 10 slices of bread in the carbohydrate count—around 225 grams!

We men love carbs, and carbs are everywhere in our favorite foods: spaghetti (or, as one nutritionist called it, "string sugar"), pizza, baked potatoes, oatmeal, broccoli, apples and grapes, Oreos, Cheerios, ice cream, candy, blueberries, strawberries, smoothies, sodas, fruit juice, watermelon, birthday cake, bagels, pierogies, yogurt, and on and on and on. Is your mouth watering yet? Sure, the carbohydrate is the macronutrient most guys reach for first.

You are well aware that too many carbs can make you fat. But what are the good-for-you carbs versus the bad-for-you ones? Carbs can be confusing, especially when you learn that "bad" carbs, eaten at specific times of day, can be very good for helping you build muscle and boost T.

Let's explore the double-edged sword of our compadre the carbohydrate.

IT'S SIMPLE— EXCEPT WHEN IT'S COMPLEX

Unlike protein and fat—which can play many roles in your body and are broken down and used for energy—carbohydrates really only serve one main purpose: to provide your body with the fuel it needs in order to function. "Carbs are your body's preferred source of energy, so eating plenty of them keeps you feeling energized and fuels your brain and your muscles during exercise," says Gidus.

Carbs come in two types: either simple or complex. Simple carbohydrates are basically sugars, made from either one or two sugar molecules. (Just a few examples include corn syrup, table sugar, brown sugar, honey, molasses, maple syrup, and candy.) Because of their simplicity, it doesn't take much effort at all for your body to process simple carbs and digest them, which can be either a good or a bad thing, depending on when you eat them.

Complex carbohydrates are made from three or more sugar molecules and are mainly found in whole plant foods (such as grains and most vegetables), as well as foods made from them (such as breads and pasta). Because of their complexity, they take a lot longer for your body to digest than simple carbohydrates.

Carbs take a lot of flak because your body turns them into one of three things: glucose (energy it needs right now), glycogen (energy it needs for later), or body fat (energy it may need way down the road).

Whenever you eat something with carbohydrates in it, your body's first job is to fill its immediate energy needs and convert some of those carbs into glucose, a sugar that gets released into your bloodstream and used for energy. It takes a certain amount of immediately accessible energy to think, move, and breathe (you know, all of those "little" functions you take for granted that your body does every day—even simply standing still). Even the minuscule amount of energy you'll need to turn to the next page is glucose-driven.

Once your body has enough glucose to go around, it begins to save it for later, turning it into glycogen, a form of glucose that's easily stored, mostly in your liver and your muscles. The glycogen stored in your liver helps fuel your brain, while the glycogen in your muscles fuels your muscles. The bonus to all that glycogen is that it also leaves your muscles looking fuller, since glycogen draws water into them, giving your muscles a harder, larger appearance without your doing a thing.

After your body has run out of room in both your liver and your muscles, that's when carbs stop becoming your friend and turn into testosterone's greatest foe. With no more room for glycogen, your body has no choice but to take whatever calories are left over from the carbs you're eating and store them as body fat.

DRINK MORE, CRAVE LESS

Staying hydrated isn't just essential for helping your body process food; it may also prevent you from overeating carbohydrates. When your body craves fluid, it will seek it from any available source. Since many carbohydrate-rich foods contain a certain degree of water, that may lead to a craving for carbs, even if your body doesn't need the extra energy, say nutritionists. And experts say that our brains often misinterpret thirst as hunger. Staying hydrated, therefore, may help your willpower when you spy a piece of whipped-cream-topped apple pie.

How Carbs Can Hurt Your T-Levels

Besides the obvious fact that consuming too many carbohydrate calories can make you fat (and less able to produce testosterone), taking the exact opposite approach to carbs by limiting them can also grind your T-levels to a screeching halt.

"You would think a great solution to the problem would simply be to drastically cut back on your carb intake altogether, but that can also backfire on testosterone," says Gidus. "Dropping your carbohydrate intake down too low only causes your body to throw many bodily functions into a lower gear, and, unfortunately for you, that means pulling back its production of testosterone."

How Carbs Can Help Your T-Levels

Picking the right types of carbs to eat, avoiding eating more than your body really needs, and ingesting them at the right times of the day can provide a steady stream of energy all day long that serves several T-friendly purposes.

One: Maintaining your blood-sugar levels at a nice, normal range can help satiate hunger without causing any sugar spikes, which can elicit an insulin response. The less insulin that is coursing through your body, the less fat your body will decide to slap on your frame without your permission.

Two: "Carbs help give you the right amount of stamina and endurance to work out at the intense level required to trigger a larger release of testosterone," says Gidus. "The more energy you can put into your workouts without running out of steam, the more you'll get back from them in terms of adding more muscle and subtracting more body fat."

Three: You need carbs to make sure your body doesn't cannibalize your hard-earned muscle for fuel. After a long night's sleep and right after your workouts, your body generally burns through most (if not all) of its glucose and glycogen. That's when your body begins to shop elsewhere for its energy, and since the only things it has access to for breaking down into glucose are your muscles and body fat, it's a flip of the coin as to how much of either one it grabs first.

"Eating carbs at these critical times can prevent your body from losing muscle tissue, which will only slow down your metabolism, make you put on more fat, and eventually tell your testes to stop making as much testosterone," says Gidus.

STRIKING A SUGAR BALANCE

As you might expect, since there are two different types of carbohydrates—simple and complex—the ways they behave in your body are different.

Every carbohydrate-based food has its own unique effect on your blood-sugar levels. Some (such as broccoli and cherries) barely make your blood-sugar levels blink, while others (like soda and pretzels) hit your sugar levels out of the park.

The way that effect is measured is called the glycemic index (GI). Every food you eat has its own individual ranking on a scale from zero to 100. Typically, scoring a higher number is a positive thing, right? Well, that's not the case with the GI. The higher a food's ranking, the faster it elevates your blood-sugar levels. That's why it's wise to get most of your carbohydrates from foods with a lower GI—that way you'll reduce your odds of elevating your blood-sugar levels and causing a surge of insulin that can cause your body to more easily store excess calories away in places that can hurt your health, your physique, and your T-levels.

GI is tested by measuring the effect on blood-sugar levels of eating exactly 50 grams of carbohydrates. Foods with a GI of 55 and below are considered low-glycemic foods, those with a GI of 70 and above are considered high-glycemic foods, and anything in between (56 through 69) is a medium-glycemic food. Most nutritionists are more focused on the first two—the low GI and high GI foods—since they typically have the biggest impact on which direction your blood-sugar levels go.

Here's a quick breakdown of some of the most basic food groups by GI:

No GI (meaning they have a zero ranking): Eggs, meats, and fish

Low GI (1–55): legumes, many fruits and vegetables (such as apples, leafy greens, and tomatoes), most dairy products, whole grains, and nuts

Medium GI (56–69): carrots, honey, oatmeal, pasta, sweet potatoes, and table sugar

High GI (70–100): white bread, rice, and most breakfast cereals, most sweetened beverages, sodas, and other drinks with added sugar

Low-glycemic foods tend to be either protein foods or complex carbohydrates that also contain a fair amount of fiber, which keeps them from evoking such a sugar surge. Because they take a lot longer to digest, they also take a lot longer to convert into glucose, producing a slower flow that keeps your blood-sugar levels even and your insulin alarm from sounding off. That steady trickle of glucose—along with the extra fiber many low-glycemic foods tend to have inside them—also leaves you feeling fuller longer during the day, so you don't end up eating more calories than your body actually needs.

High-glycemic foods tend to be simple carbohydrates, which is why they send sugar levels through the roof. Because they are almost instantaneously broken down into energy when you eat them, they overwhelm your body with glucose, making your system react by releasing fat-storing, T-diminishing insulin.

Allowing your blood-sugar levels to frequently rise and fall also creates a yo-yo effect that can confuse your body and make it crave even more carbs than it needs. To make matters even worse, high-glycemic foods also tend to be low in—if not void of—fiber, so you never quite feel full after eating them. That means that the more you eat them, the more likely you'll be coming back shortly to eat another serving to satisfy your hunger needs.

If you're confused about why a few veggies are missing from the list—such as artichokes, asparagus, broccoli, Brussels sprouts, cabbage, cauliflower, celery, cucumbers, mushrooms, onions, peppers, radishes, sugar snap peas, and tomatoes (just to name a few)—they aren't present for good reason.

Non-starchy veggies tend to be extremely low in calories, which make them very difficult to tabulate, because you would have to consume massive amounts to equal the 50 grams of carbohydrates required to measure them. For example, in order to get the GI for broccoli, you would have to eat around 19 cups of the vegetable before you reached 50 grams' worth of carbohydrate. Because that's not practical, these veggies haven't been measured and should be considered low- to no-glycemic foods.

That's the one glitch that makes the glycemic index far from foolproof. Although it's a great guide to determine the effect of most foods on your blood-sugar levels, it sometimes doesn't account for realistic portion sizes, since it's much easier to eat 50 grams' worth of carbs of one food than it is of another.

HERE'S WHERE THE FOODS MOST MEN EAT RANK ON THE GI RATING:

FRUIT

Cherries......................22
Grapefruit...................25
Prunes.......................29
Apricots (dried) 30
Apples.......................38
Pears (fresh)................38
Plums........................39
Strawberries 40
Blackberries 40
Oranges......................42
Peaches (fresh) 42
Pears (canned) 44
Grapes.......................46
Mangoes......................51
Bananas......................52
Peaches (in syrup) 52
Kiwis........................53
Apricots (fresh) 57
Papayas......................59
Pineapple (fresh) 59
Figs (dried) 61
Raisins......................64
Cantaloupe 65
Watermelon...................72
Dates 103

VEGETABLES (STARCHY)

Yams.........................37
Winter squash................41
Carrots......................47
Green peas...................48
Corn (fresh).................54
Sweet potatoes...............61
Beets........................64
Baked russet potatoes.......85
Parsnips.....................97

CEREAL

All-Bran.....................42
Raisin Bran..................61
Muesli.......................66
Cream of Wheat...............66
Special K....................69
Grape-Nuts...................71
Bran Flakes..................74
Puffed Wheat.................74
Cheerios.....................74
Shredded Wheat...............75
Corn Flakes..................81
Rice Krispies................82
Corn Chex....................83

BEANS AND PEAS

Chickpeas (dry) 28
Kidney Beans (dry)...........28
Lentils......................29
Black Beans (dry)............30
Chickpeas (canned)...........42
Black-eyed peas (canned) 42
Baked beans..................48
Kidney beans (canned)........52

JUICES

Tomato.......................38
Apple 40
Pineapple....................46
Grapefruit 48
Orange 50
Cranberry juice cocktail 68

PASTA AND GRAINS

Barley (pearled) 25
Spaghetti (whole wheat) 37
Spaghetti (white, boiled for 5 minutes)......38
Converted white rice.........38

Fettuccini...................40
Brown rice...................50
Long-grain rice..............56
Basmati rice.................58
Spaghetti (white, boiled for 20 minutes) 61
Couscous.....................65
Instant white rice 69
Risotto......................69

SUGARS

Fructose.....................19
Real maple syrup.............54
Honey 55
Sugar (sucrose)..............68
Flavored maple syrup........68

DAIRY

Plain yogurt 14
Whole milk...................27
Skim milk....................32
Fruit yogurt.................36

BREADS

Flour tortilla 30
Pumpernickel.................41
Rye..........................41
Corn tortilla 52
Hamburger bun................61
White........................70
Whole wheat (100%)...........71
Bagel........................72
Kaiser roll..................73

SOUP

Tomato.......................38
Black bean...................64
Split pea 66

Another example to illustrate that point: According to their GI ratings, artificial maple syrup (GI: 68) is actually a smarter option than eating a parsnip (GI: 97), right? But here's the thing: You only need to eat 4 tablespoons of maple syrup (about half to one-third of what the average guy squirts on his pancakes) to get 50 grams' worth of carbs, but you would have to eat 2 whole cups' worth of parsnips to get 50 grams of carbs. Which are you more likely to do—and which one are you pretty certain you'll never do? Exactly!

The point is this: For the Testosterone Transformation Diet, you'll mostly be eating low-glycemic whole foods (such as whole grains, vegetables, and

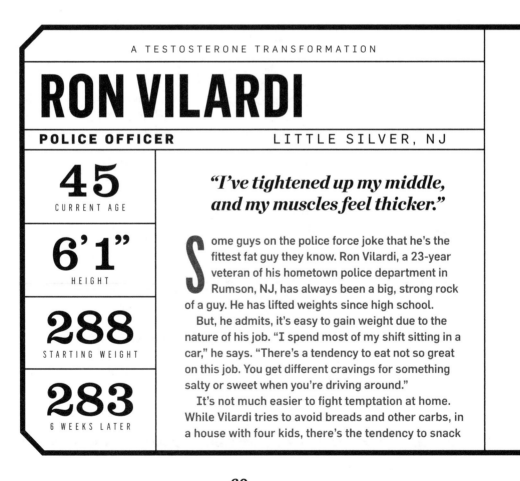

A TESTOSTERONE TRANSFORMATION

RON VILARDI

POLICE OFFICER   LITTLE SILVER, NJ

45
CURRENT AGE

6'1"
HEIGHT

288
STARTING WEIGHT

283
6 WEEKS LATER

"I've tightened up my middle, and my muscles feel thicker."

Some guys on the police force joke that he's the fittest fat guy they know. Ron Vilardi, a 23-year veteran of his hometown police department in Rumson, NJ, has always been a big, strong rock of a guy. He has lifted weights since high school.

But, he admits, it's easy to gain weight due to the nature of his job. "I spend most of my shift sitting in a car," he says. "There's a tendency to eat not so great on this job. You get different cravings for something salty or sweet when you're driving around."

It's not much easier to fight temptation at home. While Vilardi tries to avoid breads and other carbs, in a house with four kids, there's the tendency to snack fruits), in addition to some foods that may be higher on the GI list. But because you'll never be eating unrealistic portions of these high-glycemic foods, your T-levels will never be in any real danger. And remember, some of those high glycemic foods are rich in healthy vitamins and minerals. Such a mix is essential for a healthy body.

"With the T-Transformation Diet, you'll be consuming both low- and high-glycemic foods in the right proportions to provide your body with all-day energy," says Gidus. "Dual dining on carbs will also keep your muscles brimming with glycogen, so they look bigger and fuller and always have enough power to push your workouts through any plateau you may hit."

on what everyone else is eating. Vilardi saw the Testosterone Transformation test panel as a path to greater dietary discipline, weight loss, and muscle maintenance. "As I get older, I want to keep the muscle I have and add more." Plus, he has three boys to try to keep up with in the weight room.

Vilardi says the TT weight workout was similar to the weight workouts he did in his 20s but got away from in his mid 30s. "I've always been a free-weights guy, so I liked the compound exercises with barbells and dumbbells. And I've always emphasized to my boys how important it is to build a strong core and back with heavy squats and deadlifts." The volume of exercise did aggravate tendonitis, so Vilardi is planning to modify the workout, and put more emphasis on the cardio HIIT workouts to try to lose more weight.

"The meal plan was too many calories for me," Vilardi says. "For some guys, it might be right, but I can't eat that much food, so I'll reduce the number of calories and I'm sure I'll continue to lose more weight."

RESULTS: In 6 weeks, Vilardi lost 4 or 5 pounds of excess body fat—not as much as he would have hoped, but he figures the weight loss was offset by significant gains in muscle mass. "This workout had considerable impact: I feel stronger and healthier; I've tightened up my middle, and my muscles feel thicker.

"I can already feel my metabolism has increased. I have considerably more energy and I feel less tired than before starting the workouts." That means a lot to a man who juggles rotating shiftwork and finds it "nearly impossible to sleep like a normal person."

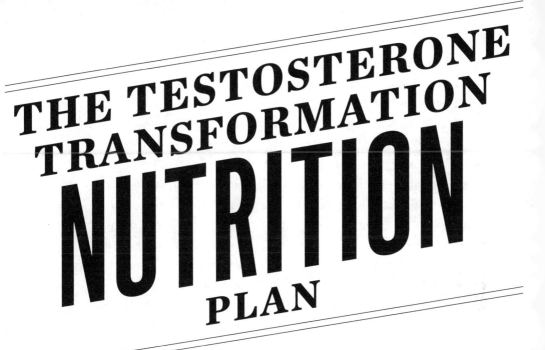

THE TESTOSTERONE TRANSFORMATION NUTRITION PLAN

Eating the right mix of macronutrients for bigger, stronger muscles

CHAPTER

08

For many people, the word diet is synonymous with the word subtract. Take away this, don't eat that. Restrict calories. Subtract fat. They subconsciously see a minus sign in front of their food.

What a depressing way to sit down to a good meal. It's no wonder most people find it extremely difficult, even impossible, to stick with a diet of denial for any length of time.

Even though we call our plan the Testosterone Transformation Diet, it has nothing to do with dieting in the traditional restrictive sense. This plan that trains you to realign your relationship with food and to "eat like an athlete."

How does an athlete think about food? Ask Gidus, the Orlando Magic's team dietitian. In a word, it's "fuel." Mealtime is gas-up time. And workouts, practice sessions, and games require athletes to time those refueling stops strategically. You will do the same on the Testosterone Transformation Plan.

"You have to eat the right number of calories to have enough energy to fuel your workouts," says Gidus. "Consuming enough calories is crucial for building muscle and keeping your body functioning properly so that it doesn't slow down testosterone production out of a belief that it's starving and needs to conserve itself."

How Many Calories Should You Eat?

The answer to that question is "Enough, but not too many." When your body doesn't get enough calories through food, your brain slows down the release of a hormone called gonadotropin-releasing hormone, or GnRH, which helps the body convert cholesterol into testosterone. For men, very low-calorie diets also reduce the activity of enzymes in the testes that accelerate testosterone production. And when you consume more calories than your body needs, you'll put on unwanted body fat—fat that triggers more enzymes to convert testosterone into the female hormone estrogen.

As you can see, it takes a balancing act to maximize testosterone through your diet. Fortunately, we have a formula to help you figure out the optimal number of daily calories to consume, considering your body composition and goals. Using math might seem like a complicated way to think about eating, but putting the right amounts of the three macronutrients into your body is as crucial to your fitness goals as the right gasoline/oxygen mixture is for optimum combustion in the engine of your Ferrari. Grab a calculator to help you figure the fat percentage and make adjustments. Once you figure out how many of your total calories should come from protein, carbs, and fat, you'll be able to plan your meals and get down to the easy part: eating.

TO ESTIMATE YOUR DAILY CALORIES, USE THIS FORMULA:

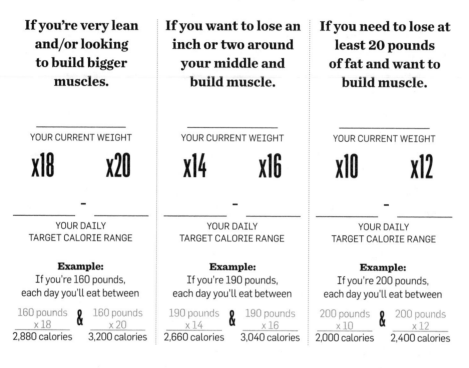

If you're very lean and/or looking to build bigger muscles.

YOUR CURRENT WEIGHT

x18   x20

-

YOUR DAILY
TARGET CALORIE RANGE

Example:
If you're 160 pounds,
each day you'll eat between

160 pounds **&** 160 pounds
x 18   x 20
2,880 calories   3,200 calories

If you want to lose an inch or two around your middle and build muscle.

YOUR CURRENT WEIGHT

x14   x16

-

YOUR DAILY
TARGET CALORIE RANGE

Example:
If you're 190 pounds,
each day you'll eat between

190 pounds **&** 190 pounds
x 14   x 16
2,660 calories   3,040 calories

If you need to lose at least 20 pounds of fat and want to build muscle.

YOUR CURRENT WEIGHT

x10   x12

-

YOUR DAILY
TARGET CALORIE RANGE

Example:
If you're 200 pounds,
each day you'll eat between

200 pounds **&** 200 pounds
x 10   x 12
2,000 calories   2,400 calories

Before you can divide up your numbers into the three macronutrients—protein, fat and carbohydrate—and start eating, you need to know four situations that may alter your daily calorie target.

1. If the high number in your daily calorie range is less than 2,000, you need a change of plan. Instead, switch to eating 2,000 calories a day. "Going lower than 2,000 calories will throw your body into starvation mode," says Gidus. "That's not pretty, for several reasons: You won't be able to build muscle, your body will end up storing more calories as fat, out of fear, and finally, your body will shut down its production of testosterone."

2. If you currently eat far more calories than your newly calculated recommended calorie range per day, gradually cut back on calories over the course of a week rather than cutting major calories all at once. Going to extremes all at once may convince your body to hoard fat. Instead, reduce consumption in 250-calorie increments every 2 or 3 days until you find yourself within your range. For example, if you usually eat 4,000 calories and now you're expected to eat 2,200 calories, start by eating 3,750 calories, then 3,500 after 2 or 3 days, and so on until you're eating the number of calories expected.

3. If you lose or gain weight during the program, recalculate your daily calorie range once a week. Don't stay in the same calorie range for the entire 12-week program unless you weigh the same as you did in the beginning, which is unlikely.

4. If you're extremely active outside of your exercise sessions—as, say, a steelworker on your feet all day at the job site—you may need to throw a few more calories into your daily target. Nutrition in the real world isn't an exact science, and that's true for eating on the Testosterone Transformation Plan. That's why we suggest a target calorie range. Use common sense to adjust the TT target calorie numbers to your personal situation. If you aren't seeing the weight loss you expect, you may need to reduce your daily food by a few hundred calories. Add calories if you want to bulk up some more.

HOW MUCH PROTEIN?

Aim to eat one gram of protein per pound of body weight per day—and that's it. Research suggests that eating more than that may actually lower your testosterone levels. Besides, eating protein in excess might supply your body with more calories than it needs, causing it to store them as fat.

Example: If you weigh 175 pounds, shoot for eating 175 grams' worth of protein daily. Since 1 gram of protein equals 4 calories, that's exactly 700 calories' worth of protein (175 grams x 4 calories = 700 calories).

HOW MANY CARBS?

Aim to eat two grams of carbohydrates per pound of body weight per day. This will create a 2:1 carbs-to-protein ratio in your diet, which has been shown to be an optimal formula for raising testosterone levels.

Example: If you weigh 175 pounds, you would eat 350 grams of carbohydrates each day. One gram of carbs, like protein, contains 4 calories, so that means you would eat around 1,400 calories' worth of carbs per day .

HOW MUCH FAT?

Twenty to 30 percent of your daily calories should come from fat—no higher. There is no "per pound of body weight" rule.

Example: If you are that 175-pound guy, you would eat 700 calories of protein and 1,400 calories of carbohydrates; adding that up gives you 2,100 calories so far. Then the remainder of your daily calories (total calories minus 2,100 protein/carb calories) would come from fat—as long as that number doesn't exceed 30 percent of your total daily calorie intake. Fat contains 9 calories per gram, so fat calories can add up fast.

Let's take a look at how the math works out for three different men who all weigh 175 pounds but have different body compositions and/or fitness goals. Grab your calculator and follow along.

....

Guy No. 1 WEIGHT: 175

GOAL: **Maintain natural leanness, looking to build muscle.**

MAX DAILY CALORIES TO EAT: 3,500 (175 pounds x 20 = 3,500)

DAILY PROTEIN: 175 grams, 700 calories (175 grams x 4 calories per gram = 700)

DAILY CARBS: 350 grams, 1,400 calories (350 grams x 4 calories per gram = 1,400)

TOTAL CALORIES FROM PROTEIN + CARBS: 2,100 (700 + 1,400 = 2,100)

FAT CALORIES (30% OF MAX DAILY CALORIES): 1,050 (.30 x 3,500 = 1,050)

TOTAL ACTUAL CALORIES FROM PROTEIN + CARBS + FAT: 3,150 (700 + 1,400 + 1,050 = 3,150)

Max daily calories (3,500) – total calories eaten (3,150) = 350 calories to spare.
Guy No. 1 falls within his 3,500-calorie goal.

....

Guy No.2 WEIGHT: 175

GOAL: **Looking to lose an inch around the waist but maintain weight, build muscle.**

MAX DAILY CALORIES TO EAT: 2,800 (175 pounds x 16 = 2,800)

DAILY PROTEIN: 175 grams, 700 calories (175 grams x 4 calories per gram = 700)

DAILY CARBS: 350 grams, 1,400 calories (350 g x 4 calories per gram = 1,400)

TOTAL CALORIES FROM PROTEIN + CARBS: 2,100 (700 + 1,400 = 2,100)

FAT CALORIES (30% OF MAX DAILY CALORIES): 840 (.30 x 2,800 = 840)

TOTAL CALORIES FROM PROTEIN + CARBS + FAT: 2,940 (700 + 1,400 + 840 = 2,940)

Following the 30-percent-fat formula, Guy No. 2 would go over his

2,800-daily-calorie max by 140 calories. (2,800 max daily calories – 2,940 actual calories = –140.)

He can eliminate the 15 fat grams (140 calories) from his diet. Another option is to drop his percentage of calories from fat to the lower end of the recommended 20–30 percent range. (Using 25 percent of calories from fat would give him exactly 2,800 calories for the day.)

Guy No.3 WEIGHT: 175

GOAL: Build muscle, lose at least 20 pounds.

MAX DAILY CALORIES TO EAT: 2,100 (175 pounds x 12 = 2,100)

DAILY PROTEIN: 175 grams, 700 calories

(175 grams x 4 calories per gram = 700 calories)

DAILY CARBS: 350 grams, 1,400 calories (

350 grams x 4 calories per gram = 1,400 calories)

TOTAL CALORIES FROM PROTEIN + CARBS: 2,100 (700 + 1,400 = 2,100) *leaves no room for fat.

FAT CALORIES (30% of max daily calories): 630 (.30 x 2,100 = 630)

TOTAL CALORIES FROM PROTEIN + CARBS + FAT: 2,730 (700 + 1,400 + 630 = 2,730)

Following the 30-percent-fat formula, Guy No. 3 would go over his 2,100-daily-calorie max by 630 calories. (2,100 max daily calories – 2,730 actual calories = –630.) He can adjust by planning to …

▶ eat 70 fewer fat grams (630 calories) or

▶ follow the low end (20 percent) of the calories-from-fat range to get daily fat calories and reduce the extra calories from carbs and protein in a 2:1 ratio. Here's what that would look like: 20 percent of 2,100 total calories is 420 calories from fat; he would reduce his carb and protein intake by 420 total calories (280 calories from carbs and 140 from protein would do it and maintain the 2:1 carb-protein ratio).

As you can see, unless you're a math whiz, a calculator comes in handy! Is this a hassle? Maybe, but remember that being able to eat exactly 1 gram of protein and 2 grams of carbs per pound of body weight, keeping your fat calories between 20 and 30 percent of total calories, and staying around your maximum daily calories is the perfect formula for maximum testosterone, according to most experts. Besides, you only have to do the calculation once to figure out how many calories or grams of each macronutrient to shoot for daily. (When your weight changes significantly, you'll recalculate.)

HOW OFTEN SHOULD YOU EAT?

"To maximize how efficiently your body burns fat all day long, you need to give your body a reason to keep your metabolism revved at an elevated pace throughout the day," says Gidus. "On the other hand, to minimize the volume of insulin your body releases (so you don't store as many excess calories as fat), you need to keep your blood sugar at a consistently low level."

The best way to accomplish both of these T-supporting tasks at once is by breaking up your calories into eight small meals that are roughly the same number of calories and eating about every 2 hours. If that seems impractical for you, I'll offer an alternative below. But first let me explain the reasons: Eating the same number of calories every 2 or 3 hours keeps your metabolism high and your sugar levels low, guaranteeing that your body always has access to energy and that your muscles are

EAT V'S TO SQUASH E'S

Mixing in some low-glycemic, cruciferous, and leafy vegetables can help you hold on to more testosterone. That's because these types of vegetables—such as broccoli, cabbage, and cauliflower—have a compound called indole-3-carbinol (I3C) that metabolizes and removes excess estrogen from your body. To keep the big E from damaging your T, try eating any of the following vegetables (raw, if you want the biggest T-protecting amount of I3C).

- ARUGULA
- BOK CHOY
- BROCCOLI
- BRUSSELS SPROUTS
- CABBAGE
- CAULIFLOWER
- COLLARD GREENS
- DAIKON
- KALE
- KOHLRABI
- RADISHES
- RUTABAGA
- TURNIP GREENS
- WATERCRESS

consistently flooded with the amino acids needed to build muscle. Second, small meals mean your body is digesting less fat at any given time. When you consume large meals that are high in fat, testosterone levels drop temporarily so your body can switch its attention from T-producing to big-meal digesting. In addition, larger meals tend to raise your stress-hormone levels, while small frequent meals keep this T killer under control.

Eight small meals strategically eaten throughout the day is the ideal way to eat for top T. That takes a little planning, thought, and discipline. But mini-meals don't have to be elaborate. A whey-protein-based fruit smoothie can be a meal. Grab a box of zip-lock bags and build mini-meals of unsalted almonds, a hardboiled egg, cheese sticks, and baby carrots to bring to work. There are dozens of ideas for simple snacks and mini-meals that'll give you the proper mix of macronutrients you're looking for. All you need to do is a little math to figure out the right number of calories for you. When you add in the whey protein drinks you'll consume before and after your workouts, it's very easy to get six to eight fuel-ups into your day.

HOW MUCH SHOULD YOU DRINK?

By now you've heard the recommendation to drink at least eight 8-ounce glasses of water a day. It's a good plan for most people, because most Americans are walking around in a constant state of dehydration, and every function in our bodies needs enough water to work properly. But eight glasses is not good enough for you if strength, muscle, and increased testosterone are your goals. We recommend double that.

Testosterone production may grind to a halt if your body isn't hydrated properly. What's more, your muscles are made up of about 75 to 80 percent water, so if you're not drinking enough of this important nutrient, your biceps won't look as big, full, and impressive in that tight black T-shirt of yours. And they won't be nearly as strong as they could be.

One classic study, published in the *Journal of Strength and Conditioning Research*, discovered that dehydration resulting in a loss of as little as 2 percent of your body weight can significantly affect both your strength and your endurance. The less energy you put into your workouts—and the less weight you're able to lift—the less testosterone your body will squeeze out as a result.

One study, out of the University of Connecticut, took seven resistance-trained men and had them perform six sets of three exercises under three different states of hydration: normal hydration, light dehydration, and significant dehydration. Researchers found that subjects' lifting performance dramatically suffered during the later sets if the men were in either state of dehydration.

As you move through the workouts in this book and improve your fitness, your water needs grow even more critical. That's because the leaner you become, the greater impact dehydration can have on your body.

We recommend you try to drink 128 ounces of water throughout the course of the day. That's 16 8-ounce glasses—and it means more trips to the men's room. But your body will love you for it.

Keep a container of ice water (a BPA-free container, that is) with you at work and sip throughout the day. On training days, weigh yourself before you begin your workout, then immediately afterwards. If the scale says you're down from where you were at the beginning of the workout, you'll need to drink exactly 1 pint (16 ounces) of water for every pound you've lost through exercise.

THE PLAN
OPTIMAL EATING EIGHT TIMES A DAY:

Most diet books—as well as many exercise books that have some type of nutritional component to them—typically provide readers with a 2- or 4-week nutritional plan that spells out exactly what to eat every day of the week. They mean well, but those types of eating plans assume you are going to have the same tastes as the writer of the book. But maybe you don't like borscht (a Russian beet soup) like I do. Maybe you are Italian and must get your weekly *pasta e fagioli* (pasta and bean soup) fix and it's nowhere to be found in your prescribed meal plan. The horror!

We're not going to try to guess your favorite dish or tell you what to eat. (You wouldn't listen to us anyway.) And we can't predict how many calories you need, because we don't know your individual weight or your personal goal. So instead, we're going to show you how to eat, with the help of sports dietitian Tara Gidus, whom you met in earlier chapters.

BREAKING DOWN THE BREAD

In the previous chapter you learned how to calculate the proper amounts of protein, carbohydrates, and fats you should be eating each day based on your goals. Now the trick is knowing how to break up those calories and grams into real meals—six to eight of them.

As mentioned earlier, you'll be eating up to eight times a day—as opposed to cramming all your calories into the traditional "three squares"—to spread your total calories more evenly over the entire course of the day. To review, the benefits of eating this way are:

▶ keeping blood-sugar levels stable to avoid insulin spikes that can lead to fat storage

▶ avoiding dips in energy so you feel alert and on top of your game all day long

▶ maintaining an elevated metabolism to burn more calories at rest (and even during sleep)

▶ allowing your muscles to absorb T-boosting amino acids for tissue repair and growth 24/7

▶ keeping your body supplied with vitamins and minerals for optimum performance of all essential organ functions

▶ providing energy and key nutrients for high-intensity workouts

Let's take the example of our 175-pound guy from earlier in this chapter who wants to lose an inch or two from his flabby belly as well as build and maintain muscle. Following the formula described in that chapter, we figured that he needed to eat close to 2,800 calories, his daily calorie maximum.

The TT Diet recommends eating 1 gram of protein and 2 grams of carbohydrates for every pound of body weight. In this case, that would give us 175 grams of protein, or 700 calories' worth, and 350 grams of carbs, or 1,400 calories' worth. That leaves 700 calories to spend on fat. You'll recall that daily fat calories should be at least 20 percent and no more than 30 percent of the total daily calories eaten. At 2,800 maximum daily calories, that gives our man between 560 and 840 calories for fat each day. So, by eating 700 calories' worth of fat (about 78 grams), he would achieve the optimal nutrition proportions for testosterone production and muscle growth.

What our guy should eat daily:

▶ **175 grams of protein**   ▶ **350 grams of carbohydrates**   ▶ **78 grams of fats**

Now, he could divide those grams by 6 to find out how much of each macronutrient he needs to eat for breakfast, lunch, dinner, and each of three snacks in between. (That would work out to 29 grams of protein, 58 grams of carbs, and 13 grams of fat at every sitting.) That'll work, and you're welcome to follow that plan. However, there are better ways.

He also could divide his total daily calories over eight meals and use a sneaky tapering trick to achieve optimal testosterone production and fat loss. Here's how it works:

First, remove the words "breakfast," "lunch," and "dinner" from your vocabulary. Most men eat more calories than necessary during those three sit-downs. Instead, you'll eat a "meal" every 2 to 3 hours.

Second, to keep your body from storing as much T-crippling body fat, taper your carbs as the day goes on. Having too many carbohydrates before bedtime only gives your body energy it doesn't need when it's about to settle down and rest, so it typically turns those calories into fat. Instead, front-load the total carbs evenly over the first six meals of the day, then slash carbs by at least 50 percent for the seventh meal. Go carb-free for the day's last meal, just before bedtime.

Bonus trick: As soon as you wake up, even before you sit down to what you used to call "breakfast" in a previous life, eat a small kick-start meal rich in simple carbohydrates, such as a half cup of watermelon or pineapple or a

MEET
TARA GIDUS, RD

DESIGNER OF THE TESTOSTERONE TRANSFORMATION DIET PLAN

Tara Gidus is one of the few registered dieticians in the country who holds board certification as a specialist in sports dietetics (CSSD). She's currently the team dietitian for the Orlando Magic NBA team, which means she's used to telling guys a lot taller and stronger than you what they should be eating in order to stay that way. So, listen up.

A former national media spokesperson for the American Dietetic Association, Gidus is a highly sought after nutrition and fitness expert for television, radio, and magazines. She appears biweekly as the "Diet Diva" on the national morning television show, *The Daily Buzz*. Gidus is owner of Tara Gidus Nutrition Consulting in Orlando, Florida. She's an active runner who has completed seven marathons.

small banana, and some easy-to-digest whey protein. Here's why: All night long, your body has been fasting, rebuilding muscle, and using up all of its spare glycogen fuel. When you wake up, your body starts hunting for fuel; without much glycogen, it may go after your muscle and cancel out the previous night's rebuilding work. This mini-meal of fast-digesting carbs quickly recharges your fuel tanks and also triggers the release of leptin, a hormone produced in your fat cells that helps regulate appetite and pull your body out of a catabolic state.

Here is how tapering your carbs and eating at eight separate times during your day plays out for our 175-pound man who wants to lose inches and build muscle:

MEAL	WHEN?	PROTEIN (grams)	CARBS (grams)	FAT (grams)	TOTAL CALORIES
MEAL 1	Immediately after you wake up	22	65	10	438
MEAL 2	One hour after Meal 1	22	55	10	398
MEAL 3	Two to three hours after Meal 2	22	60	10	418
MEAL 4	Two to three hours after Meal 3	22	55	10	398
MEAL 5	Two hours after Meal 4	22	50	10	378
MEAL 6	Two to three hours after Meal 5	22	44	10	354
MEAL 7	Two hours after Meal 6	22	21	9	253
MEAL 8	Right before bedtime	21	0	9	165
TOTALS		175 grams	350 grams	78 grams	2,800+ CALORIES

In every meal, with the exception of your first and last meals of the day, shoot to eat a mix of the following:

▶ A high-quality protein source (either through low-fat meats and dairy products or by combining grains and legumes)

▶ A complex carbohydrate (fruits, veggies, and select grains, such as oats, brown rice, or quinoa)

▶ Some form of fat, which can come from your protein source or something else, if the protein source you're eating doesn't have any (such as egg whites) **Remember:** Meal 1 is all about eating fast-digesting simple carbohydrates.

WHAT'S ON THE MENU

The beauty of the Testosterone Transformation meal plan is that it's not a diet—it's just a set of guidelines that light the way to how to eat. What you choose to eat by mixing and matching different foods is entirely up to you, so long as you eat the required number of calories for your goals, divide them up into eight small meals a day, and eat the right types of foods in each meal.

Need a few suggestions to get you going? Here are some meals that fit the bill for our example above.

SAMPLE MEALS

(for a 175-pound man looking to lose a few inches of belly and gain lean muscle)

▶ 1 cup of plain nonfat yogurt with ground flaxseed, walnuts, blueberries, and whey protein powder	▶ Turkey wrap: turkey, low-fat cheese, dark leaf lettuce, slice of avocado, tomato, and Dijon mustard on a whole-wheat tortilla	▶ 3 ounces of chicken breast, 1 ounce of raisins, and 2 ounces of walnuts
▶ 1 serving of rolled oats with ground flaxseed, walnuts, and a kiwi	▶ A large pear, 8 to 10 almonds, and 3 to 4 egg whites	▶ 3 ounces of bottom round, half cup cooked brown rice, and one cup of broccoli
▶ 1 cup of oatmeal, 3 whole eggs, 3 ounces of Canadian bacon, and one apple	▶ 2 slices of wheat bread with a tablespoon each of peanut butter and jelly, plus a glass of fat-free milk	▶ 3 ounces of pork tenderloin, 2 slices of whole-grain bread, and 1 cup of steamed snow peas

To help you figure out what's inside the foods you choose, here are some charts listing grams and calories for single portions of common proteins, carbohydrates, and fats.

PROTEIN-RICH FOODS

MEATS

	PORTION SIZE	PROTEIN (grams)	CARBS (grams)	TOTAL FAT (grams)	SATURATED FAT (grams)	CALORIES
Bacon (regular)	One slice	2	0	3	1	34
Beef tenderloin (lean, boneless, roasted)	3 ounces	24	0	6	2	152
Bison (roasted)	3 ounces	24	0	2	1	123
Bottom round (lean, roasted)	3 ounces	24	0	5	2	139
Brisket (lean, braised)	3 ounces	28	0	6	2	174
Canadian bacon	3 ounces	21	0	6	3	156
Chuck roast (lean, braised)	3 ounces	28	0	6	2	179
Eye of round (lean, roasted)	3 ounces	25	0	3	1	138
Filet mignon (lean, broiled)	3 ounces	24	0	9	3	179
Flank steak (lean, braised)	3 ounces	23	0	14	6	224
Flank steak (lean, broiled)	3 ounces	24	0	6	3	158
Ground beef (70% lean/30% fat)	3 ounces	12	0	25	9.5	279
Ground beef (80% lean/20% fat)	3 ounces	14	0	17	6.5	213
Ground beef (extra lean)	3 ounces	22	0	13	5	208
Jerky (beef)	1 ounce	9.5	3	7	3	116
Jerky (turkey)	1 ounce	15	3	0.5	0	80
Lamb chop (lean and broiled)	3 ounces	26	0	8	3	184
Pork tenderloin (roasted)	3 ounces	24	0	4	1	139
Rib steak (lean, broiled)	3 ounces	12	0	3	1	81
Roast beef (deli sliced)	3 ounces	18	3	3	3	90
T-bone steak (lean, broiled)	3 ounces	22	0	8	3	168
Top sirloin steak (broiled)	3 ounces	26	0	6	2	166
Top round steak (braised)	3 ounces	30	0	5	2	178
Veal chop (lean, braised)	3 ounces	29	0	8	2	192
Venison	3 ounces	25	0	8	2	177

PROTEIN-RICH FOODS

DAIRY

	PORTION SIZE	PROTEIN (grams)	CARBS (grams)	TOTAL FAT (grams)	SATURATED FAT (grams)	CALORIES
Cottage cheese (nonfat)	4 ounces	11	7	0	0	80
Egg (whole)	One large	6	0	5	1.5	70
Egg (white)	One large	3.6	0	0.5	0	17
Milk (whole)	1 cup	8	11.5	5	3	122
Milk (1%)	1 cup	8	12	2	1.5	102
Milk (nonfat)	1 cup	8	12	0.5	0.25	86
Yogurt (low-fat)	8 ounces	12	16	3.5	2	143
Yogurt (nonfat)	8 ounces	13	17	0.5	0.26	127

POULTRY

	PORTION SIZE	PROTEIN (grams)	CARBS (grams)	TOTAL FAT (grams)	SATURATED FAT (grams)	CALORIES
Chicken breast (boneless)	3 ounces	25	0	3	1	128
Chicken breast (with bone)	3 ounces	25	0	7	2	168
Chicken thigh (boneless)	3 ounces	21	0	8	2	166
Chicken thigh (with bone)	3 ounces	15	0	9	3	149
Duck breast (broiled)	3 ounces	23	0	2	0	119
Ostrich (ground)	3 ounces	22	0	6	2	149
Pheasant (whole)	3 ounces	28	0	10	3	210
Turkey (97% fat-free deli-sliced)	1 ounce	6	0	0	0	29
Turkey breast (roasted with skin)	3 ounces	24	0	6	2	161
Turkey dark meat (roasted with skin)	3 ounces	23	0	10	3	188
Turkey leg	3 ounces	24	0	8	3	177

PROTEIN-RICH FOODS

FISH

	PORTION SIZE	PROTEIN (grams)	CARBS (grams)	TOTAL FAT (grams)	SATURATED FAT (grams)	CALORIES
Atlantic cod (baked)	3 ounces	19	0	1	0	89
Brown trout (baked)	3 ounces	22	0	3	2	119
Carp (baked)	3 ounces	19	0	6	1	138
Catfish (steamed)	3 ounces	17	0	8	2	144
Flounder (baked)	3 ounces	21	0	1	0	100
Grouper (baked)	3 ounces	21	0	1	0	100
Haddock (baked or steamed)	3 ounces	21	0	1	0	95
Halibut (baked)	3 ounces	23	0	3	0	119
Mahimahi (baked)	3 ounces	20	0	1	0	93
Salmon (baked or broiled)	3 ounces	17	0	5	1	118
Sea bass (baked)	3 ounces	20	0	2	1	105
Sole (baked)	3 ounces	21	0	1	0	100
Striped bass (baked)	3 ounces	19	0	3	1	105
Tilapia (baked)	3 ounces	22	0	2	0	118
Trout (baked)	3 ounces	18	0	4	1	113
Tuna (canned in water)	3 ounces	20	0	3	1	109
Tuna (yellowfin; baked)	3 ounces	25	0	5	1	156

CARBOHYDRATE-RICH FOODS

FRUITS

	PORTION SIZE	PROTEIN (grams)	CARBS (grams)	FAT (grams)	CALORIES
Apple	One	0	19	0	72
Apricot (fresh or dried)	One	0	4	0	17
Banana	One (8-inch)	1	31	0	121
Blackberries	½ cup	1	7	0.5	31
Blueberries	½ cup	1	11	0	41
Cantaloupe	½ cup	0.5	7	0	13
Cherries (sour)	½ cup	1	9	0	39
Clementine	One	1	9	0	40
Cranberries	½ cup	0	6	0	22
Grapefruit	One (medium-size)	2	20	0	82
Grapes (green or red)	½ cup	1	14	0	55
Honeydew	½ cup	0.5	8	0	32
Mango	One	2	36	0	134
Nectarine	One	1	17	0	70
Orange	One (medium-size)	1	16	0	66
Papaya	½ cup	0	7	0	27
Peach	One (medium–size)	1	9	0	38
Pear	One (medium–size)	1	26	0	100
Pineapple	½ cup	0	10	0	37
Plum	One (medium–size)	0	8	0	30
Prunes	3 (medium-size)	1	13	0	50
Raisins (purple, seedless)	1 ounce	0	22	0	84
Raspberries	½ cup	0.5	8	0	32
Strawberries	½ cup	0.5	7	0	26
Watermelon	½ cup	0.5	6	0	23

CARBOHYDRATE-RICH FOODS

VEGETABLES	PORTION SIZE	PROTEIN (grams)	CARBS (grams)	FAT (grams)	CALORIES
Asparagus	4 ounces	3	5	0	25
Beets (cooked)	½ cup	1	8	0	37
Bell pepper	½ cup	0.5	5	0	20
Broccoli (steamed)	½ cup	2	4	0	22
Butternut Squash (baked)	½ cup	1	11	0	41
Cabbage (chopped)	½ cup	0.5	3	0	11
Carrot	One (medium-size)	0.5	3	0	13
Cauliflower	½ cup	1	3	0	15
Celery	½ cup	0.5	2	0	8
Corn (sweet white)	½ cup	1	8	0.5	33
Cucumber	One (8-inch)	2	11	0	45
Green Beans	½ cup	1	4	0	19
Kale	½ cup	2	4	0.5	20
Lettuce (Boston, iceberg, or romaine)	Four leaves	0 to 1	2	0	4 to 13
Peas	½ cup	4	10	4	59
Potato (baked with skin)	One medium	4	36	0	162
Snow peas (steamed)	½ cup	2	6	0	35
Spinach (cooked)	½ cup	2.5	3.5	0	20
Sweet potato (cooked and mashed)	½ cup	2	29	0	125
Tomato	One (medium-size)	1	7	1	35
Yams (cooked)	½ cup	2	18	0	78
Zucchini (steamed)	½ cup	1	3	0	13

CARBOHYDRATE-RICH FOODS

BREADS, GRAINS, AND PASTA

	PORTION SIZE	PROTEIN (grams)	CARBS (grams)	FAT (grams)	CALORIES
Angel hair pasta	1 ounce	4	21	1	102
Bagel (egg)	3 ounce	9	45	3	234
Bagel (plain)	3 ounce	9	48	0	243
Bow-tie pasta	1 ounce	4	21	1	103
Bulgur (cooked)	⅓ cup	2	11	0	50
Couscous (cooked)	⅓ cup	2	12	0	59
Pita (white)	One	6	34	0	166
Pita (whole wheat)	One	6	36	2	170
Pumpernickel	One slice	2	12	1	65
Quinoa (cooked)	⅓ cup	4	20	1	108
Rice (brown, medium, or long-grain)	⅓ cup	1.5	15	0	72
Rice (white, short-grain)	⅓ cup	1.5	17	0	80
Rye bread	One slice	3	15	1	82
Seven-grain bread	One slice	3	12	1	65
White bread	One slice	2	13	1	67
Whole-wheat bread	One slice	3	13	1	69

FAT-RICH FOODS

	PORTION SIZE	PROTEIN (grams)	CARBS (grams)	TOTAL FAT (grams)	SATURATED FAT (grams)	CALORIES
Almonds	1 ounce	6	6	14	1	164
Avocado	¼ cup	1	3	5	1	58
Butter	1 teaspoon	0	0	4	2	33
Brazil nuts	1 ounce	4	3.5	19	4	186
Cashew nuts	1 ounce	5	9	14	2.4	165
Macadamia nuts	1 ounce	2	4	21.5	3.5	204
Olive oil	1 teaspoon	0	0	5	1	40
Peanuts	1 ounce	7	4.5	14	2	161
Pecans	1 ounce	2.5	4	20.5	2	196
Pumpkin seeds (raw)	1 tablespoon	3	1	5	1	63
Sunflower seeds	1 ounce	6.5	5	14	1.5	162
Walnuts	1 ounce	4	4	18.5	2	185

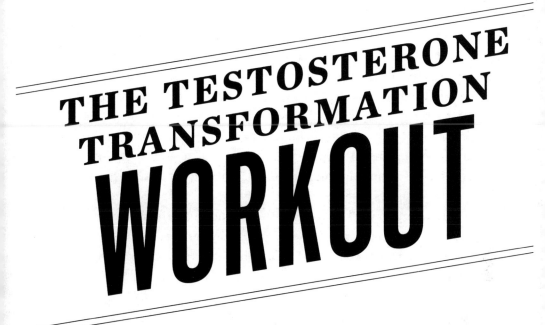

THE TESTOSTERONE TRANSFORMATION WORKOUT

The nuts and bolts of the plan and the reason why you should exercise our way

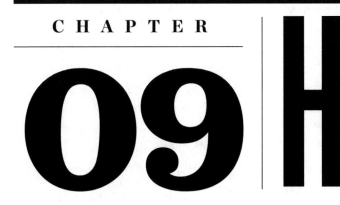

CHAPTER

09

Have you ever wondered why certain guys in the gym always seem to be bigger, stronger, more muscular, and teeming with more confidence than the rest of the pack?

It's not that they are blessed with great genetics, it's that they are using the right workout regime to get the best T-boosting results.

The guys with the most testosterone coursing through their bodies never follow the herd when it comes to lifting weights. They don't rely on traditional principles of strength training (such as sticking with performing only 3 sets of an exercise for 8 to 12 repetitions, for example). They don't waste their time on exercises that may be popular—like fitness-ball chest presses—but aren't very efficient for packing on muscle and pumping out testosterone. Instead, the taskmasters of testosterone do what you have probably never tried—namely, whatever works to get the job done, no matter how unorthodox, unconventional, or uncomfortable those tactics may be, like chest flies on a pec deck or concentration curls with a dumbbell stuck between your legs. The guys who grow lean mass and strength focus only on exercises that:

T	**E**	**S**	**T**
Turbocharge their body's natural testosterone levels	Equalize their musculature by bringing their weaker side up to speed with their stronger side so they can handle heavier weight totals when both arms or both legs work together	Shore up their core muscles so they have a more stable center, a tactic that enables them to lift even more weight than usual and yield even more testosterone than normal	Train the forgotten muscles. Most lifters ignore crucial muscles that can bullet-proof their bodies from injury so they can train harder and longer without ever needing to quit!

One of those testosterone taskmasters is strength-and-conditioning coach Josh Bryant, who designed our 12-week T-Transformation Workout.

Bryant's own transformation from skinny, inexperienced teen to record-setting powerlifter and world-class trainer (for a list of his impressive achievements, just turn to page 89) started with a simple but oft-ignored bit of advice he was given and has never forgotten.

"I was 14 the very first time I stepped into a real gym and started working with a powerlifting trainer named Steve Holl," remembers Bryant. "Before we ever got started, he sat me down and told me, "I've been in this gym for over 15 years, and I've seen a lot of these same faces every day, lifting the exact same weights in the exact same way—and in all that time, none of them have ever changed one bit. Don't ever fall into that trap,' he said."

Although that was many years ago, Bryant can still hear Holl's advice in his head as if it was yesterday. It's a talk he now gives to his clients—and it's the impetus behind the Testosterone Transformation Workout.

"Even if you have the time and dedication to get in shape, the most common mistake that causes men to fail is sticking with a program long after their body has already adapted to its intensity." In other words, don't fall into a rut, especially the "3 sets of 8 to 12 repetitions rut." You're about to experience a paradigm shift, thanks to Bryant and the power of change.

FROM A TRICKLE TO A TIDE

Getting your body to release more testosterone requires focusing on five separate muscle areas. Fortunately for you, the Testosterone Transformation Workout you're about to undertake mixes all five in the same plan, so you're guaranteed to send your T-levels through the roof each and every week you're on the program.

1. MUSCLE MATH

"Your body releases a certain volume of anabolic hormones—such as testosterone—that's relative to the intensity of a workout," says Bryant. More work = more T. But it takes pushing your body hard enough to make it happen, something that most lifters don't accomplish. Still, you can do it in many ways, including:

▶ lifting the heaviest weights possible while maintaining safe
▶ overloading your muscles with a greater volume of sets than they are used to doing
▶ giving your body little time to rest during exercise
▶ activating as many muscle fibers as possible at once

That last bullet point is why the backbone of the T-Transformation Workout relies on a series of compound exercises that target your largest muscle groups (your back, quadriceps, hamstrings, and chest). These moves are designed to recruit as many muscle fibers as possible as efficiently as possible.

The foundation of the T-Transformation Workout is composed of the squat, the deadlift, and the bench press, three of the most valuable compound exercises you can use if maximum testosterone is your goal. Each of these classic, old-school exercises "requires your body to involve hundreds of muscles—including prime movers that lift the weight, secondary movers that assist with the lift, and stabilizer muscles that keep your body centered as you perform the lift," says Bryant. "Because of all that work, all three exercises have been shown to cause a greater spike in testosterone, growth hormone, and other anabolic hormones than most other exercises."

Count your weight loads: Another proven way to stimulate the greatest release of testosterone and other anabolic hormones is to overload your muscles. The squat, bench, and deadlift also are ideal exercises for accomplishing this. Using these primary moves with the other exercises in the workouts, you'll find your strength rising every week, as demonstrated by the increasing weight load you'll be able to heft.

Count your reps, sets, and the seconds in between: Remember the 3-sets-of-12 rut we told you to break out of? Here's why it's a bad place to be if your goal is more T. Research has shown that performing five sets of an exercise can significantly increase blood levels of testosterone. Other studies have indicated that performing low repetitions using heavy weights (about 70 to 85 percent of your one-repetition max) can also raise your T-levels. Why? Both boost the intensity of the exercise. What's more, using shorter rest periods between sets can also trigger the body to release extra testosterone (as well as growth hormone). All three of these tactics help exhaust your muscles more thoroughly, which forces your body to cough up even more testosterone than usual.

Our workout plan delivers all of this: low-rep, heavy-weight exercises; high-rep, light-weight exercises; higher-than-typical set volumes; and shorter rest intervals between sets. This way the Testosterone Transformation Workout hits a variety of rep ranges that force your body to activate both slow-twitch and fast-twitch muscle fibers within the same workout.

PAY ATTENTION FOR MORE PAYOFF

Details make the difference in the Testosterone Transformation Workout. Here are four key points:

1 TERMINOLOGY

Know the vocabulary. You already know that *rep* is short for repetition. A set is a group of repetitions. For example, doing 1 set of 10 repetitions means you'll need to perform the exercise 10 times consecutively.

2 PUSH YOURSELF HARD

For each exercise, you start with a weight that lets you perform the required number of repetitions. Odds are, you'll choose a weight load that's too light for you on the first try. When researchers at Grand Valley State University, in Allendale, Michigan, asked subjects to pick weights they thought were heavy enough for them to exercise with, all of them chose weights that were lighter than what they should have been using. That's fine, so long as you make sure to adjust accordingly.

If you can't do the recommended number of repetitions, then the weight is too heavy, so lower the weight you're using until you find the right amount. If you can do more repetitions than what's recommended, then the weight is too light, so increase the weight.

As you get stronger, you'll need to increase the amount of weight you're using to keep your muscles challenged. You can do that by raising the weight by between half a pound and 5 pounds, depending on the exercise and what you feel you can handle.

3 PAY ATTENTION TO THE NUMBERS

Unlike many standard workouts in which you're asked to do 3 sets of an exercise for 8 to 12 repetitions, you may be asked to do up to 8 sets of a particular exercise—or as little as 1 set. You may be asked to do 1 repetition with as much weight as you can handle or do as many as 30 repetitions using a lighter weight. Keeping a close eye on the numbers will ensure that you don't do too much or too little, in order to see maximum results.

4 BUY A STOPWATCH

The time you spend resting between sets is just as crucial to boosting testosterone as the exercises you're performing, so don't take it lightly—count every second. The amount of time you'll rest between sets will vary from as little as 30 seconds to as much as 180 seconds. If the rest interval reads "as needed," that means you can rest up until you feel ready to do another set. However, try not to take too much advantage of this rest period—5 minutes is the maximum time your body should require.

NOTE: You'll see "as needed" only on the heaviest and most difficult, multi-muscle, compound exercises.

Which twitch, you ask? Muscles are made up to two different types of fibers. The first, slow-twitch (Type I) fibers, contract at a very slow speed, which allows them to take much longer to fatigue. This makes them the muscle fiber of choice for all low-intensity, long-duration movements you make—from standing to walking to doing many reps of weight loads that are 70 percent or less of your maximum effort. These are high-resistance fibers—the marathon fiber, if you will.

Fast-twitch (Type II) fibers contract at a much faster pace, which makes them more efficient at generating short bursts of force, speed, or strength. The only problem: They burn out a lot faster as well. That's why your body turns to them only during high-intensity, short-duration movements, such as jumping, sprinting, or lifting weight loads that are more than 70 percent of your maximum effort. These are the explosive fibers, the sprinter variety.

Your muscles are generally split 50/50 between the two types. Many guys never bother training their Type I muscle fibers using higher repetitions and lighter-weight exercises, because they know Type II muscle fibers are capable of producing greater force, which allows them to grow much more effectively and evoke a greater testosterone reaction. But that's a mistake. Type I fibers still have the ability to grow up to 15 to 20 percent, so training both can maximize your muscle-growth potential. That's one reason we target Type I fibers in this workout, too.

From a strictly testosterone-boosting perspective, adding a few high-repetition, lighter-weight exercises serves two purposes. One: It allows you to train more muscle fibers. Two: It can help flush excess lactic acid from your muscles. Lactic acid is the chemical by-product left in muscles that's responsible for the burning sensation you sometimes feel after intense exercise. Having less of this stuff in your muscles will leave you feeling fresher immediately after each workout, instead of sore.

2. MUSCLE TENSION

Too many men count reps and sets, and a few of the smart ones even pay attention to the time between each exercise, but the ones who see the biggest boost in T also pay attention to how long their muscles stay under continuous stress.

Certain exercises in this program help achieve optimal release of testosterone and muscle growth by utilizing the "time under tension" (TUT) principle, the idea that the longer your muscles remain contracted to resist a weight load during exercise, the better for T production.

For example, most guys will stick with the tried-and-true 2-seconds-up, 2-seconds-down rule of thumb when raising a weight. If you perform 8 repetitions, that means the TUT range for your muscles is 32 seconds (4 seconds per rep times 8 reps). However, take those same 8 repetitions and force yourself to raise or lower the weight at a much slower pace (say, 8 seconds per rep) and the TUT your muscles experience doubles—even though you've performed the same number of reps.

So what does that have to do with testosterone? Easy. When you apply this high-intensity technique to your workout, your muscles spend even more time in a contracted state, which helps them activate even more fibers than usual. This, in turn, elevates the amount of damage you impose on your muscles. Because you're breaking down more fibers, your muscles are forced to rebuild themselves to be bigger and stronger, which can help pack on even greater muscle volume in a

MEET JOSH BRYANT

DESIGNER OF THE TESTOSTERONE TRANSFORMATION WORKOUT

Strength-and-conditiong coach Josh Bryant is a rising star in the fitness training industry. He's a world-record-holding powerlifter, founder of the JoshStrength Method (www.joshstrength.com), and a trainer at the famed Metroflex Gym, in Arlington, Texas.

In addition to being an NSCA-certified strength-and-conditioning specialist and NASM-certified performance-enhancement specialist, Bryant also holds a master's degree in exercise science, with an emphasis on performance enhancement and injury prevention. He was recently named the ISSA director of applied strength and power development.

Bryant has won several national and world titles in both powerlifting and strongman competitions, including the Atlantis Strongest Man in America competition in 2005. He trained powerlifters, women's fitness competitors, Olympic athletes, professional fighters, and NCAA champions.

shorter amount of time—especially if you're new to the method.

But more important to T-seekers is how using TUT also causes your body to secrete higher levels of testosterone, growth hormone, and other important hormones at the end of your workout, giving your entire body a muscle-building boost!

What sets the Testosterone Transformation Workout apart is that it utilizes the TUT principle beyond what you might expect, especially for guys looking for the complete package from their muscles—size, strength, and stamina. If that's your Holy Grail, then incorporating exercises that place your muscles under a mix of TUT ranges—between 4 and 30 seconds for strength; 30 to 60 seconds for size; and 60-plus seconds for stamina—is key. The T-Transformation Workout does exactly that!

3. MUSCLE CONFUSION

Once your muscles get used to an exercise routine, they begin to figure out how to do the same movements more efficiently. That may sound like a plus in theory, but it's a problem if what you're hoping for is more testosterone and better overall results.

As your muscle adapts to an exercise, less muscle damage occurs. That's the big reason most guys plateau with their workouts, either by seeing less muscle building up and less body fat burning off, or by failing to see any results at all. The way to keep your muscles from adapting—from, in essence, getting lazy—is to keep them confused. The Testosterone Transformation Workout keeps your muscles guessing by changing up the mix of supportive exercises every four weeks. You'll keep doing your main big-muscle moves, like the deadlift, squat, and bench press, but you'll be introduced to new exercises that will keep your muscles from becoming too familiar with the routine.

Each new mix of exercises alters the type of resistance you'll use (from barbells to dumbbells to body-weight moves) and brings in training variables like lifting tempo, muscular-contraction type, and arm and leg position. When combined in one workout, these exercises make it virtually impossible for your muscles to fall into a rut. Plus, every subtle tweak lets you utilize a different ratio of muscle fibers. The more variations you use in the same workout, the more muscle fibers you'll exhaust, which will result in a greater release of testosterone.

4. MUSCLE PROTECTION

Training for big muscle isn't easy, especially because in order to induce the type of hormonal response you're gunning for, you have to push your body to its limits. The downside of that hard work is the stress on certain areas—specifically your hips, lower back, and shoulders.

Bryant's program incorporates functional exercises, such as scapular retractions, clamshells, and shoulder boxes, that are designed to keep your muscle healthy. Most of these moves might seem unexciting, but they are crucial to your ability to go harder, longer, without risking injury. Each of the functional exercises in the T-Transformation Workout serves a purpose, ranging from preventing your shoulders from rounding forward by realigning your scapular stabilizers to strengthening your external hip rotators to prevent back pain and help support your knees.

All these tiny corrections have the same effect as the little things a mechanic might do when tuning up your car. By adding these oft-neglected exercises into the program, you'll be far less likely to break down halfway through.

THE RIGHT REP SPEED TO RAKE IN MORE T!

To ensure that you'll train as many muscle fibers as possible, Bryant's program incorporates a series of exercises that are performed at various rep speeds. "Both slower and faster rep speeds stimulate your muscle fibers in different ways," says Bryant. "The more variety you employ in your exercise routine, the more muscle fibers you'll exhaust in each workout."

Unless noted in the exercise description, take 1 to 2 seconds to raise the weight and 1 to 2 seconds to lower it.

However, when performing exercises using heavy weight for low reps (6 or fewer), it may take longer to raise the weight (between 3 and 4 seconds), while the lowering portion may take less time, due to gravity taking over and your muscles fatiguing as you continue through the set.

Perform exercises using lighter weight and higher reps (12 or more), as explosively as possible when raising the weight, then lower the weight under control for a count of 1 to 2 seconds. This technique—known as compensatory acceleration training—allows your muscles to generate more power and recruit more muscle fibers than they typically would at a normal 2-seconds-up pace.

5. MUSCLE MAXIMIZATION

A chain is only as strong as its weakest link. And when it comes to being able to lift the greatest amount of weight, your body is only as strong as its weakest muscles. For most guys looking for maximum testosterone, that weak link is front and center—meaning the core muscles.

All of your power goes through your torso, which means that the stronger your abs and core muscles are, the more stability and power you'll have during the multijoint exercises that elicit the greatest testosterone response. That's why the Testosterone Transformation Workout incorporates a series of special core-stabilization exercises that turn your weakest link into your strongest asset.

But that weak-link maxim doesn't end with your midsection—it can also occur when one side of your body is weaker than the other. Most of the multijoint exercises that generate the greatest testosterone release are bilateral exercises that require either both of your arms, both legs, or your entire body to raise and lower a weight. The problem: Whenever you reach exhaustion, it's typically your weaker side (say, your left, if you're a righty) that fails first.

Throughout our workout, you'll perform specific unilateral exercises that ask you to train one arm or one leg at a time. It's a tactic that can help eliminate any muscular imbalances in your physique by bringing your weaker arm or leg up to speed with your dominant one—an improvement that will make a noticeable difference in how much weight you can handle during bilateral exercises.

There's a bonus benefit to unilateral training that few men even consider: All of the best T-boosting multijoint exercises require a certain degree of coordination—the more in sync your muscles are with your mind, the more stable you'll be when performing them. The more stable you are, the less energy your body has to waste trying to maintain balance. That's energy it could be transporting into the exercise to lift more weight and summon forth even more testosterone. Working one side at a time can help speed up how quickly you're able to forge the mind-muscle connection needed for balance movements.

BLAST-OFF BASICS

Ready to start pumping big iron? Hold on. Before you launch your T-levels into the stratosphere using Bryant's 12-week program, you need to know the ground rules—and if you're a guy who has been lifting for a while and thinks he can skip this basics chapter, then this chapter is written especially for you.

The very reason you're reading this book is because the workouts you've been using until now haven't built the kind of muscle you were looking for. What might have held you back in past workouts may be as simple as warming up improperly, resting too long between sets, or not following a few other simple steps in this chapter that really should be old habit for a seasoned lifter like you.

It's time to forget what you think you know so your T-levels can finally grow.

The Official T-Template

In order to shoot a spacecraft into Earth's orbit, it typically takes a three-stage rocket to generate enough propulsion to break through gravity's grip. What you're about to use to launch your T-levels skyward and beyond takes a similar three-stage approach.

The 12-week program that Bryant designed is a 4-day-a-week routine, broken up into three stages: three 4-week programs. You'll perform each stage to the letter, right down to the amount of time required to rest between sets.

"Do not perform all four workouts one after another during the week—your muscles need time to recover from each workout," says Bryant. Instead space them out in either of the following schedules.

MONDAY	**Day 1**		**MONDAY**	**Day 1**
TUESDAY	**Rest**	**OR**	**TUESDAY**	**Day 2**
WEDNESDAY	**Day 2**		**WEDNESDAY**	**Rest**
THURSDAY	**Rest**		**THURSDAY**	**Day 3**
FRIDAY	**Day 3**		**FRIDAY**	**Day 4**
SATURDAY	**Rest**		**SATURDAY**	**Rest**
SUNDAY	**Day 4**		**SUNDAY**	**Rest**

As you perform each stage, you'll notice a gradual increase in intensity from weeks 1 through 3. When you reach the 4th week of each stage, you'll notice that the exercises change slightly and the intensity decreases.

There's a reason for this three-steps-forward, one-step-back approach. "One of the biggest mistakes most men make with weight training is thinking they need to constantly raise the bar each and every week to reach their goals," says Bryant. "That mindset is the reason most guys never see results in the first place, since it only leads to overtraining and a higher risk of injury."

This high-intensity, multi-angled routine is so effective because it is so exhausting on your body, muscles, and central nervous system. "Giving yourself a break on the 4th week of each stage will give your muscles and central nervous system sufficient time to recover—leaving you feeling fresher and stronger to start the next stage," says Bryant.

You'll also notice that you'll be training certain muscles less often during the week than traditional workout routines recommend. This may feel counterproductive, but the extreme effort of these programs requires a once-a-week approach to targeting specific muscle groups—a strategy that will allow you to experience faster and more substantial results.

Avoid Aerobic Activity

That's right. For best results, you must resist the temptation to do extracurricular activities such as pickup basketball, football, running, cycling, swimming, skipping rope—basically anything that might put additional stress on your body or prevent it from getting enough rest. Done in the traditional slow and long style, aerobic exercise can cannibalize your muscles and send your T-levels right into the toilet. When have you ever seen an elite cyclist or marathon runner with hulky muscles? You see our point: These guys are fit, but usually thin. They don't pack on muscle because their training methods stifle muscle growth.

Long-duration aerobic exercise—say, running five miles—definitely has its benefits when it comes to strengthening your heart. But research has shown that long bouts of aerobic exercise undermine testosterone production and muscle growth by overtraining your body and causing it to lose weight too quickly. According to a Finnish study, dropping pounds at a rapid pace can cause your body to significantly turn down testosterone production. When researchers looked at the effects of a 2- to-3-week weight-reduction regimen on 18 elite wrestlers, they found that those who lost weight quickly experienced significant dehydration and decreased testosterone and other hormone concentrations. Feeling fatigued from too much cardio can hamper your weight-training workouts, preventing you from lifting enough weight or with enough intensity. That's why rest and recovery are so crucial to muscle size. If you do the Testosterone Transformation Workout as prescribed, you'll get plenty of good exercise for your heart and blast away fat, too.

However, if you are eager to fry even more fat or if you simply love to run, we have an option for you: Instead of long-and-steady aerobic workouts, do a brief but intense interval workout. High-intensity interval training, or HIIT, is any short aerobic workout that alternates between quick bursts of high effort and short low-intensity recovery periods. For example, instead of setting the treadmill at one speed for 45 minutes, run on that treadmill at an all-out pace for 8 seconds, then jog or walk at an easy pace for 12 seconds, and repeat the cycle for 20 minutes.

The work intensity of HIIT forces your body to burn through glycogen, its easy-access fuel, and start burning fat much sooner than with long, slow aerobics. In a study in the *Journal of Applied Physiology*, volunteers who performed seven HIIT sessions over a 2-week period experienced a 20 percent increase in their muscle mitochondria, and their fat oxidation increased 36 percent.

The Testosterone Transformation HIIT Workout

A 2011 study at the University of Nebraska-Lincoln tested four different HIIT programs of different intensities and durations. The researchers found that the most effective workout for improving fitness was a HIIT program that entailed switching back and forth between high-intensity exercise (performed at 90 percent of maximum effort) for 30 seconds and low-intensity exercise for 30 seconds.

Our optional TT HIIT workout follows a similar time-and-intensity pattern. First, choose your favorite aerobic activity: running, cycling, skipping rope, and even walking up and down stadium stairs.

▶ Start with a 5-minute low-intensity warm up.

▶ Set your sports watch to beep at 30-second intervals, and then begin sprinting for 30 seconds. Your effort level should be between 7 and 9, where

10 represents your absolute maximum effort. (At a 7- to -9-intensity pace, you can speak short phrases but anything longer would be impossible.)

▶ At the beep, immediately slow down to a low-intensity recovery pace for 30 seconds. (Your intensity should be between 3 and 5; you can talk with a little effort but couldn't sing.)

▶ Keep repeating that cycle 20 times for a 20-minute workout, and you're done. For the first few weeks of the Testosterone Transformation program, do your HIIT workout just once a week. Eventually you can bump it up to twice a week, spaced a few days apart. The ideal times to do HIIT: either right after your resistance workout or first thing in the morning on an empty stomach. It's during these two times that you'll burn the greatest amount of fat.

(If you're time crunched, try our shorter, even easier HIIT workout in Chapter 12, on page 129.)

Warm Up Before the Countdown

Each stage—and every exercise—works together to make sure the release of testosterone you experience is titanic. But not preparing your body in the right way before you exercise can sink your efforts before you even begin. Doing some type of light activity prior to each workout will help bring blood into your muscles to make them more pliable, so you're less likely to pull them and injure yourself.

Even if your muscles have plenty of blood flowing through them, doing a warmup set before certain exercises (using less weight than you plan to lift for the duration of the exercise) provides your muscles with a "testing ground" that lets them know what you're about to ask of them. You see, any time you perform an exercise, your muscles have to spend a little time remembering the flow of the movement in order to do it correctly. The problem is that all of that adjusting requires energy—energy that, if spent during a working set, might prevent you from moving as much T-boosting weight.

To make your muscles promise to put forth everything they've got, stay true to these T-sparing rules:

Before each workout

Warm up your muscles by doing light, low-intensity cardio for five minutes, such as jogging in place or riding the stationary cycle in a low gear.

HOW TO FIND YOUR 1-REP MAX

hoosing the right amount of weight to lift for any medium-to-higher-rep exercise in this book (moves that ask you to perform 8 repetitions or more) is easy, since it should only take a single workout to determine through trial and error which amount of weight is right for you for each exercise. That's why you won't find recommendations on how much weight to lift to start—trust us, after one session you'll learn very quickly whether you need to grab a 20-, 30-, or 40-pound dumbbell to do a biceps curl.

Before beginning the 12-week Testosterone Transformation program, determine your 1-rep max (1RM), or the maximum weight that you can lift with proper form for only 1 repetition. You'll need to know this weight in order to load the bar properly when performing such exercises as bench press, squat, and deadlift requiring 8 or fewer repetitions.

THERE ARE TWO WAYS TO DO THIS:

1 Load a bar with a weight that you know you can do, say, 10 times and then gradually add weight until you find a load that you can lift only once. Warning: Always use a spotter when using this method.

2 A much easier, safer approach: First determine how much weight you can lift with proper form for 10 repetitions, then divide that number by 0.75. For example, if you can bench-press 175 pounds for 10 repetitions, then your estimated 1RM for the bench press would be 233 pounds (175 ~ 0.75 = 233). Once you have that number, you can use it to figure out how much weight you should be using for any exercise throughout the 12-week program that requires you to lift a percentage of your 1-rep max.

"This isn't a perfect science," says Bryant. "You may be able to lift more, or need to lift less, depending on your own muscular make-up, but it's a solid starting place that can keep you from wasting sets by using too much or not enough weight."

Before any exercise that calls for low reps

Do an extra warmup practice set. For exercises requiring 8 or fewer repetitions, warm up with lighter weights to prepare your muscles for the main lift. (Note: Your warmup sets should never be volume sets, i.e. doing a lot of repetitions with much lighter weight. This will only rob your muscles of strength they could be spending during your heaviest lifts. Instead, do only enough reps to prepare your muscles for the movement.)

The purpose of this practice warmup set is to activate muscle memory so that your muscles are ready and stable enough to execute the heavy main lift properly without exhausting your muscles before the main working set.

Here's how to do this warmup right:

A) Perform the exercise using just the bar (or, if using dumbbells, a weight that's roughly 10 to 15 percent of your 1-rep max in that exercise) and do 5 to 10 reps.

B) Change the weight to 30 to 35 percent of your 1-rep max and do 3 reps.

C) Change the weight to 45 to 50 percent of your 1-rep max and do 3 reps.

D) Finally (and this is only if the exercise requires you to do 1 or 2 reps preset), load up a weight that's around 70 to 75 percent of your 1-rep max and do 1 rep.

Example (deadlift): If your 1-rep maximum for the deadlift is 300 pounds—and you're being required to do a few sets of the deadlift for 1 rep each—before you start that first working set, here's how you'll warm up:

A) Start with an empty bar—an Olympic version that weighs 45 pounds—and do the exercise 5 to 10 times.

B) Add a 25-pound plate to each side (95 pounds) and do 3 reps.

C) Add another 25-pound plate to each side (145 pounds) and do 3 reps.

D) Load the bar so that it weighs 225 pounds and do a single rep.

E) Perform the working exercise as recommended in the routine.

Instead of feeling fried at the end of each warmup, your muscles will be fresh. You'll instantly find yourself handling even more weight than usual with proper form when performing all of the power exercises that matter most—the perfect game plan for overloading your muscles for the greatest T boost.

READ YOUR FATIGUE TO SPARE YOUR T!

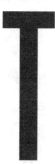he 12-week program you're about to embark on is rigorous, so you need to watch out for overtraining and ensure that you are able to recover from workouts. Overtrain, and you run the risk of hitting a plateau that can increase your risk of injury, weaken your immune system, and put the brakes on results.

Your body responds to overtraining by decreasing the amounts of testosterone, growth hormone, and other anabolic hormones it produces as it simultaneously increases the amount of cortisol in your system.

▶ Do you find yourself getting sick often?

▶ Do you find yourself not able to complete several workouts in a row?

▶ Are you experiencing any chronic joint pain?

▶ Do you feel lethargic, irritable, or drained?

▶ Is your resting heart rate more elevated than normal? (Before you start the workout, take your pulse the moment you wake up for the first few days to get a baseline number. As you perform the 12-week routine, your resting pulse rate each morning should never rise any higher than seven extra beats per minute. If it does, you may be overtraining.)

Although the Testosterone Transformation Workout is a high-intensity program, it's designed to escalate at a pace that will give your body time to acclimate to it. It's also set up with just the right amount of recovery time between workouts. However, we can't account for everything. Is your body already exhausted from a previous workout routine? Are you coming off an illness? Have you been burning the candle at both ends with work and social activities? All these can limit the effectiveness of this program and, worse, set you up for injury.

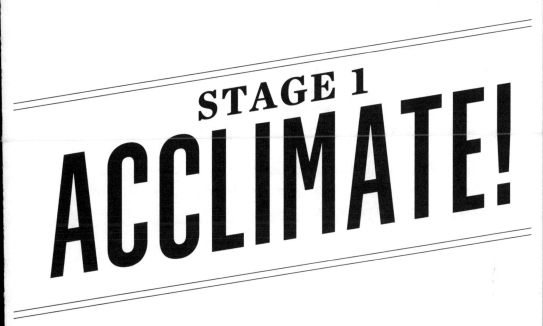

STAGE 1
ACCLIMATE!

Prime your muscles with strategic lifting during the first 4 weeks

C H A P T E R

10

W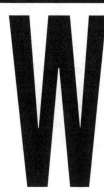elcome to the first 4 weeks of the Testosterone Transformation Workout, a three-stage progression that will turbocharge your T-levels.

Trainer Josh Bryant (see page 89) calls this the Acclimation Stage. It's during these first few weeks that your body will begin to acclimate to the exercises and the increased exertion from high-volume lifting. But if you're thinking that you'll have to wait until you complete all three stages to experience the T-level surge you're looking for, you'll be happy to hear that's not the case.

Starting with the very first workout, you'll train your body at the right intensity using the perfect combination of multijoint, multimuscle moves, and you'll apply the best rep, set, and rest principles to evoke the greatest testosterone response.

Stage 1 is the single most important stage, because it's the phase that will decide whether you truly have what it takes to build big muscle. The first 3 weeks of the Testosterone Transformation Workout are definitely the most difficult. Not only will you be exercising at an accelerated intensity you might not be used to, but you'll also be performing certain movements that require more coordination, core strength, and concentration than your average routine. Your rest breaks between all the primary lifts—the squat, the bench press, and the deadlift—will also be shorter than during the other two stages.

Stage 1 is hard for a reason. "The problem with many lifting programs is that they don't establish a base of fitness," says Bryant. "Trying to do a series of exotic exercises before building any type of muscular foundation puts you at risk of injury and limits your overall strength potential."

In the 4th week, you'll perform what Bryant refers to as a "deload" week, in which you'll exercise at less intensity using less weight. The reasoning for easing up a bit is simple: "Lifting heavy weights in the way you'll perform them in this routine will tax your central nervous system considerably," says Bryant. Dialing back your efforts will allow your body to recover—not just your muscles but your central nervous system as well—so you avoid over-training and lower your risk of injury.

"The guideline to follow is exercise at about 70 percent of your total intensity during the deload week," says Bryant. "So if you're using 100 pounds for an exercise during the first 3 weeks of the program, you'll switch to using 70 pounds—70 percent of the weight—during the 4th and final week of the stage."

Here's the best part. "Don't be surprised if you find yourself gaining the most muscle during your deload week," says Bryant. "The routine is designed to beat up your body during the first 3 weeks to elevate your T-levels, so when it's allowed to recover on the 4th week, you open up an anabolic window that gives your body the opportunity to return to normal, so you'll end up feeling healthier, stronger, and less winded for starting Stage 2."

Extra T Tools!

For maximum testosterone, you'll need a few other pieces of equipment besides access to heavy weights—barbell, dumbbells, etc.—and a chinup bar. Three unorthodox tools of the trade for Stage 1 are an old truck tire, a sledgehammer, and a training sled.

If using these types of equipment sounds extreme, you're right: They're extremely effective at helping your body produce copious amounts of testosterone! That's why athletes in the know, ranging from strongmen to mixed martial artists, swear by them to deliver high-T results, explosive strength, and massive muscle. Don't worry; none of this gear will break the bank. You can snag a free truck tire at almost any tire store or local garage, and didn't your uncle Joe use an old sledgehammer to break up the sidewalk when he replaced it last summer? (Hunt for a 4-to-6-pound hammer. The strongest of men can use a heavier sledge, but don't go over, say, 18 pounds.)

A Prowler (a.k.a. Lung Breaker) training sled is a flat sheet of metal that holds weight plates, sandbags, or rocks (or anything heavy). By connecting one end of a rope to the sled and the other end to yourself—via a belt or a set of handles—you can pull the sled across a flat surface, such as grass, a gym floor, or a track or macadam. Training sleds can cost as little as $50 and as much as $200, but it's one of the best investments you will ever make when training for testosterone. (Know someone with an acetylene torch? You can weld your own sled out of angle iron and some sheet metal.) Due to the high-intensity effort required to perform sled drags and pushes, your body's response is a greater release of testosterone and growth hormone. But better still, these exercises also help you increase your speed, reaction time, strength, and explosiveness. In the gym, that advantage can help pre-condition your muscles to withstand longer, more intense workouts, which can lead to a boost in testosterone.

Sled training also makes an impact on your overall functional strength by teaching your arms, legs, and core muscles to work together. It's an advantage that makes your body better at stabilizing itself during squats, deadlifts, lunges, and other multijoint, muscle-building exercises—so you're able to lift heavier weight loads.

The Stage 1 Workout

As mentioned in the last chapter, you should weight-train 4 times a week using one of the sample schedules on page 106 to ensure adequate recovery periods. Start each workout by performing a quick 5-minute warmup to loosen up your joints. You can cycle in a low gear, perform a light jog in place, or do any low-intensity activity that pumps blood into your muscles to prime them for action.

Once you're warmed up, perform each exercise listed in the chart below for the recommended reps and sets before moving on to the next exercise. Continue working your way through each exercise in the exact order presented in the chart, resting for the recommended number of seconds between each set. These workouts contain more exercises (as well as more sets) than you may be used to performing in a single workout, so allot yourself enough time. Each workout will take 60 to 75 minutes to complete. You'll find all the exercise descriptions and photographs in Chapter 13.

NOTE: One thing you'll see at the start of certain days is that a primary exercise, such as the bench press and the deadlift, may be repeated twice in the chart. That's not a mistake—you'll be performing these primary moves twice, but in two different ways. The first is a more intense version in which you will lift heavier weight loads for fewer repetitions (in order to take advantage of your muscles while they are at their freshest).

"That's why the rest intervals are 'as needed,'" says Bryant, "For these sets, you'll be going balls-out, whereas for the second version of the exercise you'll be performing more repetitions and using about 65 to 70 percent of the maximum amount of weight you could normally handle."

Going heavy first also engages your nervous system to recruit as many muscle fibers as possible. The perk to this—beyond releasing the maximum amount of testosterone—is that when you lower the weight to perform the second version, your nervous system will still tend to recruit the same maximum amount of muscle fibers that it called upon during the first, heavier version, letting you enjoy the same max-fiber benefit without needing to lift as much weight.

For any unilateral exercises (where you're asked to train one arm or one leg at a time), you'll notice that the exercise descriptions insist that you start by training your non-dominant arm or leg first. You always want to train your weaker side first, when your energy levels are fresh, and your dominant side second, when you are more tired.

Do a HIIT, If You Wish

Remember, our optional High Intensity Interval Training workout described on page 95. You may wish to do this speedy aerobic workout once a week, if you are looking to burn more fat. You'll find another, even quicker HIIT workout described on page 129.

ACCLIMATE

WEEK 1

DAY 1

Exercise	Rest Interval	REPS	SETS
BENCH PRESS	As needed	3	2
(FOR SET 1, TRY 75% OF YOUR 1RM; FOR SET 2, TRY 80% OF YOUR 1RM)			
BENCH PRESS	60 seconds	6	4
(FOR ALL SETS, TRY 65% OF YOUR 1RM)			
INCLINE PRESS	90 seconds	6	4
INCLINE FLY / PUSHUP SUPERSET	60 seconds	12/max	4
(MAX OUT YOUR PUSHUP SET)			
CHINUP	90 seconds	5 (if you can do more, add weight)	5
SINGLE-ARM ECCENTRIC BARBELL CURL	90 seconds	3	5
INCLINE DUMBBELL CURL	60 seconds	10 reps each/30 reps total	3
INCLINE I-Y-T	60 seconds	10 reps each/30 reps total	3
HANGING KNEE RAISE	45 seconds	15	3
ISO PRONE AB	45 seconds	60 seconds	3

DAY 2

Exercise	Rest Interval	REPS	SETS
SQUAT	As needed	5	5
(FOR ALL SETS, TRY 75% OF YOUR 1RM)			
FRONT SQUAT	90 seconds	12	2
(FOR ALL SETS, TRY 50% OF YOUR 1RM FOR A REGULAR SQUAT)			
WALKING 45-DEGREE PLATE LUNGE	60 seconds	20 yards	3
LEG CURL	60 seconds	12	4
LEG EXTENSION	45 seconds	30	3
SINGLE-LEG GLUTE BRIDGE	30 seconds	12	3
MINI-BAND CLAMSHELL	30 seconds	10	3
STANDING PLATE TWIST	45 seconds	10	5
CALF RAISE	45 seconds	20	5
BARBELL COMPLEX	180 seconds	10	3
HANGING KNEE RAISE	45 seconds	12	3
HANGING LEG RAISE	45 seconds	9	3

DAY 3

Exercise	Rest Interval	REPS	SETS
STANDING OVERHEAD PRESS	As needed	8	3
(FOR ALL SETS, TRY 65% OF YOUR 1RM)			
LATERAL RAISE AND HOLD	90 seconds	30 seconds	3
SHOULDER BOX	60 seconds	10	3
REAR DELTOID FLY	45 seconds	12	3
LATERAL RAISE SUPERSET	60 seconds	20 seconds	3
PAUL DICKS PRESS	90 seconds	12	4
DECLINE CLOSE-GRIP BENCH PRESS	75 seconds	15	3
(EZ-CURL BAR)			
TRICEPS KICKBACK	45 seconds	10	3
HANGING KNEE RAISE	45 seconds	15	3
SIDE ISO AB	45 seconds	40 seconds	3

DAY 4

Exercise	Rest Interval	REPS	SETS
DEADLIFT	As needed	3	2
(FOR SET 1, TRY 70% OF YOUR 1RM; FOR SET 2, TRY 80% OF YOUR 1RM)			
DEADLIFT	60 seconds	4	6
(FOR ALL SETS, TRY 65% OF YOUR 1RM)			
DUMBBELL SHRUG	60 seconds	10	5
YATES ROW	60 seconds	8	4
DUMBBELL PULLOVER	75 seconds	12	3
STRAIGHT-ARM PULLDOWN	45 seconds	12	4
WEIGHTED CHINUP 21	45 seconds	21	2
SINGLE-ARM DUMBBELL ROW	45 seconds	12	3
SLEDGEHAMMER	75 seconds	Maximum	3
(MAXIMUM REPS EACH WAY FOR 30 SECONDS)			
SLED DRAG	60 seconds	20 yards	6
HANGING KNEE RAISE	45 seconds	12	3
SPREAD V LEG RAISE	45 seconds	6	3

WEEK
2

DAY 1

Exercise	Rest Interval	REPS	SETS
BENCH PRESS	As needed	3	2
(FOR SET ONE, TRY 78% OF YOUR 1RM; FOR SET TWO, TRY 83% OF YOUR 1RM)			
BENCH PRESS	60 seconds	8	4
(FOR ALL SETS, TRY 65% OF YOUR 1RM)			
INCLINE PRESS	90 seconds	8	4
INCLINE FLY SUPERSET MAX PUSHUP	60 seconds	12/max	4
CHINUP	90 seconds	5	5
SINGLE-ARM ECCENTRIC BARBELL CURL	90 seconds	3	5
INCLINE DUMBBELL CURL	60 seconds	12	3
INCLINE I-Y-T	60 seconds	12	3
HANGING KNEE RAISE	45 seconds	15	3
ISO PRONE AB	45 seconds	65 seconds	3

DAY 2

Exercise	Rest Interval	REPS	SETS
SQUAT	As needed	5	5
(FOR ALL SETS, TRY 80% OF YOUR 1RM)			
FRONT SQUAT	90 seconds	10	2
(FOR ALL SETS, TRY 55% OF YOUR 1RM FOR A REGULAR SQUAT)			
WALKING 45-DEGREE PLATE LUNGE	60 seconds	25 yards	3
LEG CURL	60 seconds	14	4
LEG EXTENSION	45 seconds	50, 30, 20	3
SINGLE-LEG GLUTE BRIDGE	30 seconds	13	3
MINI-BAND CLAMSHELL	30 seconds	11	3
STANDING PLATE TWIST	45 seconds	10	5
CALF RAISE	45 seconds	20	5
BARBELL COMPLEX	180 seconds	8	3
HANGING KNEE RAISE	45 seconds	12	3
HANGING LEG RAISE	45 seconds	9	3

DAY 3

Exercise	Rest Interval	REPS	SETS
STANDING OVERHEAD PRESS	As needed	6	4
(FOR ALL SETS, TRY 70% OF YOUR 1RM)			
LATERAL RAISE AND HOLD	90 seconds	35 seconds	3
SHOULDER BOX	60 seconds	12	3
REAR DELTOID FLY	45 seconds	14	3
LATERAL RAISE SUPERSET	60 seconds	20 seconds	3
PAUL DICKS PRESS	90 seconds	10	4
DECLINE CLOSE-GRIP BENCH PRESS	75 seconds	20, 15, 12	3
(EZ-CURL BAR)			
TRICEPS KICKBACK	45 seconds	12	3
HANGING KNEE RAISE	45 seconds	15	3
SIDE ISO AB	45 seconds	50 seconds	3

DAY 4

Exercise	Rest Interval	REPS	SETS
DEADLIFT	As needed	3	2
(FOR SET 1, TRY 75% OF YOUR 1RM; FOR SET 2, TRY 80% OF YOUR 1RM)			
DEADLIFT	60 seconds	4	8
(FOR ALL SETS, TRY 65% OF YOUR 1RM)			
DUMBBELL SHRUG	60 seconds	12	5
YATES ROW	60 seconds	9	4
DUMBBELL PULLOVER	75 seconds	14	3
STRAIGHT-ARM PULLDOWN	45 seconds	15	4
WEIGHTED CHINUP 21	120 seconds	21	2
SINGLE-ARM DUMBBELL ROW	60 seconds	12	3
SLEDGEHAMMER	75 seconds	Maximum	3
(MAXIMUM REPS EACH WAY FOR 40 SECONDS)			
SLED DRAG	60 seconds	20 yards	8
HANGING KNEE RAISE	45 seconds	12	3
HANGING SPREAD V LEG RAISE	45 seconds	8	3

ACCLIMATE

DAY 1

Exercise	Rest Interval	REPS	SETS
BENCH PRESS	As needed	3	2
(FOR SET 1, TRY 80% OF YOUR 1RM; FOR SET 2, TRY 85% OF YOUR 1RM)			
BENCH PRESS	60 seconds	10	4
(FOR ALL SETS, TRY 65% OF YOUR 1RM)			
INCLINE PRESS	90 seconds	10	4
INCLINE FLY / PUSHUP SUPERSET	60 seconds	12/max	4
(MAX OUT THE PUSHUP SET)			
CHINUP	90 seconds	5	5
SINGLE-ARM ECCENTRIC BARBELL CURL	90 seconds	5	5
INCLINE DUMBBELL CURL	60 seconds	8	3
INCLINE I-Y-T	60 seconds	15	3
HANGING KNEE RAISE	45 seconds	15	3
ISO PRONE AB	45 seconds	65 seconds	3

DAY 2

Exercise	Rest Interval	REPS	SETS
SQUAT	As needed	5	5
(FOR ALL SETS, TRY 85% OF YOUR 1RM)			
FRONT SQUAT	90 seconds	8	2
(FOR ALL SETS, TRY 60% OF YOUR 1RM FOR A REGULAR SQUAT			
WALKING 45-DEGREE PLATE LUNGE	60 seconds	30 yards	3
LEG CURL	60 seconds	14	4
LEG EXTENSION	45 seconds	25	3
SINGLE-LEG GLUTE BRIDGE	30 seconds	14	3
MINI-BAND CLAMSHELL	30 seconds	12	3
STANDING PLATE TWIST	45 seconds	10	5
CALF RAISE	45 seconds	20	5
BARBELL COMPLEX	180 seconds	7	3
HANGING KNEE RAISE	45 seconds	12	3
HANGING LEG RAISE	45 seconds	9	3

DAY 3

Exercise	Rest Interval	REPS	SETS
STANDING OVERHEAD PRESS	As needed	5	5
(FOR ALL SETS, TRY 80% OF YOUR 1RM)			
LATERAL RAISE AND HOLD	90 seconds	45 seconds	3
SHOULDER BOX	60 seconds	14	3
REAR DELTOID FLY	45 seconds	15	3
LATERAL RAISE SUPERSET	60 seconds	20 seconds	3
PAUL DICKS PRESS	90 seconds	8	4
DECLINE CLOSE-GRIP BENCH PRESS	75 seconds	10	3
(EZ-CURL BAR)			
TRICEPS KICKBACK	45 seconds	15	3
HANGING KNEE RAISE	45 seconds	15	3
SIDE ISO AB	45 seconds	50 seconds	3

DAY 4

Exercise	Rest Interval	REPS	SETS
DEADLIFT	As needed	3	2
(FOR SET 1, TRY 80% OF YOUR 1RM; FOR SET 2, TRY 85% OF YOUR 1RM)			
DEADLIFT	60 seconds	4	10
(FOR ALL SETS, TRY 65% OF YOUR 1RM)			
DUMBBELL SHRUG	60 seconds	15	5
YATES ROW	60 seconds	8	4
DUMBBELL PULLOVER	75 seconds	15	3
STRAIGHT-ARM PULLDOWN	90 seconds	12	5
WEIGHTED CHINUP 21	90 seconds	21	2
SINGLE-ARM DUMBBELL ROW	90 seconds	15	3
SLEDGEHAMMER	75 seconds	Maximum	3
(MAXIMUM REPS EACH WAY FOR 45 SECONDS)			
SLED DRAG	60 seconds	20 yards	10
HANGING KNEE RAISE	45 seconds	12	3
HANGING SPREAD V LEG RAISE	45 seconds	8	3

ACCLIMATE

DAY 1

Exercise	Rest Interval	REPS	SETS
BENCH PRESS	60 seconds	5	3
INCLINE PRESS	60 seconds	10	3
INCLINE FLY	60 seconds	12	3
CHINUP	60 seconds	5	3
SINGLE-ARM ECCENTRIC BARBELL CURL	60 seconds	5	3
INCLINE DUMBBELL CURL	60 seconds	8	2
INCLINE I-Y-T	60 seconds	8	2
HANGING KNEE RAISE	60 seconds	15	3
ISO PRONE AB	60 seconds	65 seconds	3

DAY 2

Exercise	Rest Interval	REPS	SETS
SQUAT	60 seconds	5	3
FRONT SQUAT	60 seconds	8	2
WALKING 45-DEGREE PLATE LUNGE	60 seconds	20 yards	2
LEG CURL	60 seconds	14	2
LEG EXTENSION	60 seconds	20	2
SINGLE-LEG GLUTE BRIDGE	60 seconds	10	2
MINI-BAND CLAMSHELL	60 seconds	8	2
STANDING PLATE TWIST	60 seconds	10	3
CALF RAISE	60 seconds	20	3
BODYWEIGHT LUNGE	60 seconds	Max reps for 30 seconds	2
HANGING KNEE RAISE	60 seconds	12	3
HANGING LEG RAISE	60 seconds	9	3

DAY 3

Exercise	Rest Interval	REPS	SETS
STANDING OVERHEAD PRESS	60 seconds	5	5
LATERAL RAISE AND HOLD	60 seconds	30 seconds	3
SHOULDER BOX	60 seconds	14	3
REAR DELTOID FLY	60 seconds	15	3
LATERAL RAISE	60 seconds	12	3
PAUL DICKS PRESS	60 seconds	8	4
DECLINE CLOSE-GRIP BENCH PRESS (EZ-CURL BAR)	60 seconds	10	3
TRICEPS KICKBACK	60 seconds	15	3
HANGING KNEE RAISE	60 seconds	15	3
SIDE ISO AB	60 seconds	50 seconds	3

DAY 4

Exercise	Rest Interval	REPS	SETS
DEADLIFT	60 seconds	3	3
DUMBBELL SHRUG	60 seconds	15	3
YATES ROW	60 seconds	8	3
DUMBBELL PULLOVER	60 seconds	10	2
STRAIGHT-ARM PULLDOWN	60 seconds	12	3
SINGLE-ARM DUMBBELL ROW	60 seconds	8	2
SLED DRAG	60 seconds	20 yards	5
HANGING KNEE RAISE	60 seconds	12	3
HANGING SPREAD V LEG RAISE	60 seconds	8	3

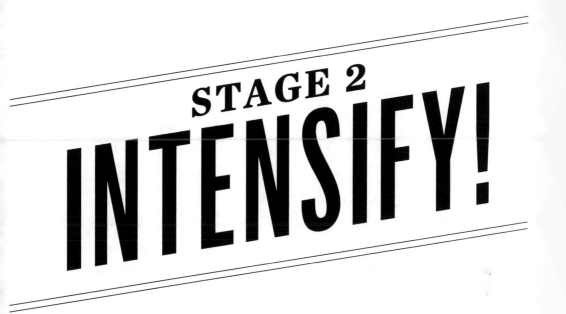

INTENSIFY!

A 4-week muscle-overload workout program

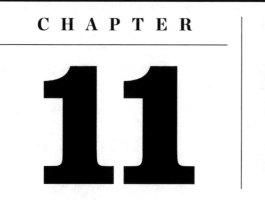

CHAPTER

11

B

y now—4 weeks in—you should already feel like a different man. You're not sore anymore. You're stronger, more skilled at performing these exercises (so you're ready to lift heavier weight), and your body has been pumping out more of the stuff that separates the men from the boys. You've now reached what Bryant refers to as "the intensification phase," because your body is ready to be tested with intense lifts that require you to give everything you've got. Although the primary lifts are still in place, many of the original core-stabilizing, multijoint, and isolation exercises are gone, replaced by challenging new exercises designed to keep your muscles guessing—and growing.

More Tools For Extra T!

You should already have three important tools from Stage 1 that you'll need for Stage 2: an old tire, a sledgehammer, and a training sled. However, there are a few new pieces of equipment you'll be adding to your muscle arsenal for the next 4 weeks.

The first is four 12- to 18-inch-long pieces of 2-by-6-inch wood. Pine is fine. In two of the exercises in this stage—the Three-Board Press and the Close-Grip Burnout—you'll have a training partner place boards on your chest to limit your range of motion as you press the weight up and down. "Overloading your muscles with partial movements this way will elevate your strength potential when performing the same exercise during a full range of motion," says Bryant. "The more weight you can handle, the greater the T-boost you can expect."

If you don't have access to boards, you can also use pieces of Styrofoam that are roughly the same size. (But expect to have to replace them often because of all the wear and tear.)

The second tool you need is an ab wheel, a $5 exercise device that looks like a lawnmower wheel with bike-grip-like handles sticking out on both sides. Typically, it's used by grabbing an end in each hand, getting on all fours on the floor, and rolling it forward as far as possible before using your core muscles to roll yourself back. However, for our workout, you'll use it to do a unique hand-walking exercise that Bryant prefers because it engages even more of your core, plus your chest, shoulders, and triceps.

Finally, you'll need a large tractor-trailer tire to perform the Tire Flip, an old-school strongman exercise for building T-surging explosive power.

"You may think a big tire is impossible to find or too expensive," says Bryant, "but the truth is, it costs the businesses that handle used tires a lot of money to dispose of them, so expect them to beg you to take them off their hands." Just call any tire center, and if they don't have one to give away, they can usually direct you to a place that does.

The Stage 2 Workout

Begin each workout in Stage 2 with a quick 5-minute warmup to loosen up your joints.

Once you're warmed up, perform each exercise for the recommended reps and sets before moving on to the next exercise in the chart. Continue working your way through each exercise in the exact order presented in the chart, resting for the recommended number of seconds between each set. You'll do four of these resistance-training workouts a week, according to one of the sample schedules on page 118. Each workout will take you roughly 60 to 75 minutes.

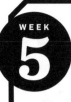
INTENSIFY

DAY 1

Exercise	Rest Interval	REPS	SETS
BENCH PRESS	As needed	2	2
(FOR SET 1, TRY 85% OF YOUR 1RM; FOR SET 2, TRY 90% OF YOUR 1RM)			
BENCH PRESS	75 seconds	5	4
(FOR ALL SETS, TRY 70% OF YOUR 1RM)			
THREE-BOARD PRESS	90 seconds	6, 4, 3	3
(FOR SET 1, TRY 85% OF YOUR 1RM; FOR SET 2, TRY 90% OF YOUR 1RM; FOR SET 3, TRY 95% OF YOUR 1RM)			
BOTTOM END DRIVE	90 seconds	6	2
SINGLE-ARM INCLINE DUMBBELL PRESS	60 seconds	15, 10, 8, 8	4
STANDING CABLE FLY	45 seconds	15	3
SCAPULAR RETRACTION	45 seconds	12	3
CHINUP	120 seconds	8, 6, 3, 10	4
CHEAT CURL	90 seconds	10, 8, 7, 6	4
ZOTTMAN CURL RACK RUN	120 seconds	8	1
BICEPS SLED CURL	120 seconds	30 yards	2
AB WHEEL HAND WALKING	45 seconds	10 yards	3
ISO PRONE AB	45 seconds	75 seconds	3

DAY 2

Exercise	Rest Interval	REPS	SETS
SQUAT	As needed	4	2
(FOR SET 1, TRY 82% OF YOUR 1RM; FOR SET 2, TRY 87% OF YOUR 1RM)			
SQUAT	75 seconds	4	4
(FOR ALL SETS, TRY 75% OF YOUR 1RM)			
ZERCHER SQUAT	90 seconds	12	2
BULGARIAN ISOMETRIC SQUAT	120 seconds	45 seconds	2
LATERAL LUNGE	60 seconds	12	2
GLUTE BRIDGE	60 seconds	6	4
SINGLE-LEG PRESS	60 seconds	20, 15, 10	3
SINGLE-LEG GLUTE BRIDGE	30 seconds	12	3
MINI-BAND CLAMSHELL	30 seconds	10	3
STANDING PLATE TWIST	45 seconds	10	5
CALF RAISE	45 seconds	20	5
BARBELL COMPLEX	120 seconds	10	3
LAND MINE	45 seconds	10	3
HANGING WINDSHIELD WIPER	45 seconds	12	3

DAY 3

Exercise	Rest Interval	REPS	SETS
STANDING OVERHEAD PRESS	As needed	6	3
(FOR ALL SETS, TRY 83% OF YOUR 1RM)			
SEATED MILITARY PRESS	As needed	5	3
(OVERLOAD) (FOR ALL SETS, TRY 95% OF YOUR 1RM)			
ARNOLD PRESS	90 seconds	Max 30 seconds	3
SHOULDER BOX	60 seconds	12	3
FLAT-BENCH REVERSE FLY	45 seconds	12	3
LATERAL T-RAISE	60 seconds	25, 15, 8, 20	4
JM PRESS	90 seconds	8	4
CLOSE-GRIP BURNOUT	180 seconds	25	2
SINGLE-ARM TRICEPS CABLE PUSHDOWN	45 seconds	15	3
DIAMOND PUSHUP	60 seconds	Max 30 seconds	1
HANGING KNEE RAISE	45 seconds	15	3
SIDE ISO AB	45 seconds	55 seconds	3

DAY 4

Exercise	Rest Interval	REPS	SETS
DEADLIFT	As needed	2	2
(FOR SET 1, TRY 84% OF YOUR 1RM; FOR SET 2, TRY 90% OF YOUR 1RM)			
DEADLIFT	75 seconds	3	6
(FOR ALL SETS, TRY 73% OF YOUR 1RM)			
TRAP-BAR SHRUG	90 seconds	20, 15, 10, 30, 30	5
T-BAR ROW	90 seconds	15, 12, 6, 12	4
DUMBBELL PULLOVER	75 seconds	15	3
FARMER'S WALK	90 seconds	20 yards	3
WEIGHTED CHINUP	150 seconds	3	4
45-DEGREE BENT-OVER ROW	60 seconds	15	5
SLEDGEHAMMER	75 seconds	Maximum	3
(MAXIMUM REPS EACH WAY FOR 50 SECONDS)			
TIRE FLIP	60 seconds	16 yards	5
SIDE MEDICINE-BALL TOSS	45 seconds	12	3
DECLINE BENCH REVERSE CRUNCH	45 seconds	10	3

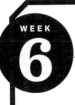

INTENSIFY

DAY 1

Exercise	Rest Interval	REPS	SETS
BENCH PRESS	As needed	2	2
(FOR SET 1, TRY 82% OF YOUR 1RM; FOR SET 2, TRY 92% OF YOUR 1RM)			
BENCH PRESS	75 seconds	5	5
(FOR ALL SETS, TRY 73% OF YOUR 1RM)			
THREE-BOARD PRESS	90 seconds	5, 4, 2	3
(FOR SET 1, TRY 85% OF YOUR 1RM; FOR SET 2, TRY 94% OF YOUR 1RM; FOR SET 3, TRY 103% OF YOUR 1RM)			
BOTTOM END DRIVE	90 seconds	6	2
SINGLE-ARM INCLINE DUMBBELL PRESS	60 seconds	12, 10, 8, 6	4
STANDING CABLE FLY	45 seconds	15	3
SCAPULAR RETRACTION	45 seconds	12	3
CHINUP	120 seconds	6, 5, 3, max body weight	4
CHEAT CURL	90 seconds	10, 8, 6, 5	4
ZOTTMAN CURL RACK RUN	120 seconds	10	1
BICEPS SLED CURL	120 seconds	40 yards	2
AB WHEEL HAND WALKING	60 seconds	15 yards	3
ISO PRONE AB	45 seconds	75 seconds	3

DAY 2

Exercise	Rest Interval	REPS	SETS
SQUAT	As needed	3	2
(FOR SET 1, TRY 85% OF YOUR 1RM; FOR SET 2, TRY 92% OF YOUR 1RM)			
SQUAT	75 seconds	4	4
(FOR ALL SETS, TRY 77% OF YOUR 1RM)			
ZERCHER SQUAT	90 seconds	12	2
BULGARIAN ISOMETRIC SQUAT	120 seconds	55 seconds	2
LATERAL LUNGE	60 seconds	12	2
GLUTE BRIDGE	60 seconds	8	4
SINGLE-LEG PRESS	60 seconds	20, 15, 10	3
SINGLE-LEG GLUTE BRIDGE	30 seconds	12	3
MINI-BAND CLAMSHELL	30 seconds	10	3
STANDING PLATE TWIST	45 seconds	10	5
CALF RAISE	45 seconds	20	5
BARBELL COMPLEX	120 seconds	9	3
LAND MINE	45 seconds	10	3
HANGING WINDSHIELD WIPER	45 seconds	12	3

DAY 3

Exercise	Rest Interval	REPS	SETS
STANDING OVERHEAD PRESS	As needed	5	3
(FOR ALL SETS, TRY 86% OF YOUR 1RM)			
SEATED MILITARY PRESS	As needed	5	3
(OVERLOAD; FOR ALL SETS, TRY 100% OF YOUR 1RM)			
ARNOLD PRESS	90 seconds	Max 40 seconds	3
SHOULDER BOX	60 seconds	14	3
FLAT-BENCH REVERSE FLY	45 seconds	13	3
LATERAL T-RAISE	60 seconds	20, 12, 6, 30	4
JM PRESS	90 seconds	7	4
CLOSE-GRIP BURNOUT	180 seconds	25	2
SINGLE-ARM TRICEPS CABLE PUSHDOWN	45 seconds	15	3
DIAMOND PUSHUP	45 seconds	Max 40 seconds	1
HANGING KNEE RAISE	45 seconds	15	3
SIDE ISO AB	45 seconds	55 seconds	3

DAY 4

Exercise	Rest Interval	REPS	SETS
DEADLIFT	As needed	2	2
(FOR SET 1, TRY 90% OF YOUR 1RM; FOR SET 2, TRY 95% OF YOUR 1RM)			
DEADLIFT	75 seconds	3	7
(FOR ALL SETS, TRY 75% OF YOUR 1RM)			
TRAP-BAR SHRUG	60 seconds	20, 15, 12, 12, 20	5
T-BAR ROW	60 seconds	15, 12, 6, 12	4
DUMBBELL PULLOVER	75 seconds	12	3
FARMER'S WALK	90 seconds	20 yards	3
WEIGHTED CHINUP	150 seconds	3	4
45-DEGREE BENT-OVER ROW	60 seconds	15	5
SLEDGEHAMMER	85 seconds	Maximum	3
(MAXIMUM REPS EACH WAY FOR 55 SECONDS)			
TIRE FLIP	60 seconds	16 yards	5
SIDE MEDICINE-BALL TOSS	45 seconds	12	3
DECLINE BENCH REVERSE CRUNCH	45 seconds	12	3

INTENSIFY

DAY 1

Exercise	Rest Interval	REPS	SETS
BENCH PRESS	As needed	2	2
(FOR SET 1, TRY 87% OF YOUR 1RM; FOR SET 2, TRY 96% OF YOUR 1RM)			
BENCH PRESS	75 seconds	5	6
(FOR ALL SETS, TRY 73% OF YOUR 1RM)			
THREE-BOARD PRESS	90 seconds	3, 2, 1	3
(FOR SET 1, TRY 90% OF YOUR 1RM; FOR SET 2, TRY 100% OF YOUR 1RM; FOR SET 3, TRY 105% OF YOUR 1RM)			
BOTTOM END DRIVE	90 seconds	6	2
SINGLE-ARM INCLINE DUMBBELL PRESS	60 seconds	10, 8, 6, 5	4
STANDING CABLE FLY	45 seconds	15	3
SCAPULAR RETRACTION	45 seconds	12	3
CHINUP	120 seconds	4	4
CHEAT CURL	90 seconds	8, 6, 5, 5	4
ZOTTMAN CURL RACK RUN	120 seconds	12	1
BICEPS SLED CURL	180 seconds	50 yards	2
AB WHEEL HAND WALKING	45 seconds	20 yards	3
ISO PRONE AB	45 seconds	75 seconds	3

DAY 2

Exercise	Rest Interval	REPS	SETS
SQUAT	As needed	3	2
(FOR SET 1, TRY 88% OF YOUR 1RM; FOR SET 2, TRY 95% OF YOUR 1RM)			
SQUAT	75 seconds	4	5
(FOR ALL SETS, TRY 77% OF YOUR 1RM)			
ZERCHER SQUAT	90 seconds	8	2
BULGARIAN ISOMETRIC SQUAT	120 seconds	60 seconds	2
LATERAL LUNGE	60 seconds	12	2
GLUTE BRIDGE	60 seconds	9	4
SINGLE-LEG PRESS	60 seconds	16, 14, 12	3
SINGLE-LEG GLUTE BRIDGE	30 seconds	12	3
MINI-BAND CLAMSHELL	30 seconds	10	3
STANDING PLATE TWIST	45 seconds	10	5
CALF RAISE	45 seconds	20	5
BARBELL COMPLEX	120 seconds	9	3
LAND MINE	45 seconds	10	3
HANGING WINDSHIELD WIPER	45 seconds	12	3

DAY 3

Exercise	Rest Interval	REPS	SETS
STANDING OVERHEAD PRESS	As needed	4	4
(FOR ALL SETS, TRY 90% OF YOUR 1RM)			
SEATED MILITARY PRESS	As needed	5	3
(OVERLOAD) (FOR ALL SETS, TRY 105% OF YOUR 1RM)			
ARNOLD PRESS	90 seconds	Max 50 seconds	3
SHOULDER BOX	60 seconds	15	3
FLAT-BENCH REVERSE FLY	45 seconds	14	3
LATERAL T-RAISE	60 seconds	10, 8, 6, 20	4
JM PRESS	90 seconds	6	4
CLOSE-GRIP BURNOUT	180 seconds	25	2
SINGLE-ARM TRICEPS CABLE PUSHDOWN	45 seconds	15	3
DIAMOND PUSHUP	45 seconds	Max 45 seconds	1
HANGING KNEE RAISE	45 seconds	15	3
SIDE ISO AB	45 seconds	60 seconds	3

DAY 4

Exercise	Rest Interval	REPS	SETS
DEADLIFT	As needed	2	2
(FOR SET 1, TRY 90% OF YOUR 1RM; FOR SET 2, TRY 100% OF YOUR 1RM)			
DEADLIFT	75 seconds	3	8
(FOR ALL SETS, TRY 75% OF YOUR 1RM)			
TRAP-BAR SHRUG	60 seconds	30	4
T-BAR ROW	60 seconds	10, 8, 5, 12	4
DUMBBELL PULLOVER	75 seconds	12	3
FARMER'S WALK	90 seconds	20 yards	3
WEIGHTED CHINUP	150 seconds	4	4
45-DEGREE BENT-OVER ROW	60 seconds	15	5
SLEDGEHAMMER	90 seconds	Maximum	3
(MAXIMUM REPS EACH WAY FOR 60 SECONDS)			
TIRE FLIP	60 seconds	20 yards	5
SIDE MEDICINE-BALL TOSS	45 seconds	12	3
DECLINE BENCH REVERSE CRUNCH	45 seconds	15	3

DAY 1

Exercise	Rest Interval	REPS	SETS
BENCH PRESS	60 seconds	5	3
THREE-BOARD PRESS	60 seconds	5	2
BOTTOM END DRIVE	60 seconds	6	2
SINGLE-ARM INCLINE DUMBBELL PRESS	60 seconds	8	2
STANDING CABLE FLY	60 seconds	15	2
SCAPULAR RETRACTION	60 seconds	12	3
CHINUP	60 seconds	5	3
SEATED CABLE CURL	60 seconds	10	3
ZOTTMAN CURL	60 seconds	12	3
AB WHEEL HAND WALKING	60 seconds	10 yards	3
ISO PRONE AB	60 seconds	75 seconds	3

DAY 2

Exercise	Rest Interval	REPS	SETS
SQUAT	60 seconds	5	2
ZERCHER SQUAT	60 seconds	6	2
BULGARIAN ISOMETRIC SQUAT	60 seconds	30 seconds	1
LATERAL LUNGE	60 seconds	12	2
GLUTE BRIDGE	60 seconds	8	2
SINGLE-LEG PRESS	60 seconds	10	2
SINGLE-LEG GLUTE BRIDGE	60 seconds	12	3
MINI-BAND CLAMSHELL	60 seconds	10	3
STANDING PLATE TWIST	60 seconds	10	5
CALF RAISE	60 seconds	20	5
BARBELL COMPLEX	120 seconds	6	2
LAND MINE	60 seconds	10	3
HANGING WINDSHIELD WIPER	60 seconds	12	3

DAY 3

Exercise	Rest Interval	REPS	SETS
STANDING OVERHEAD PRESS	60 seconds	5	2
ARNOLD PRESS	60 seconds	12	2
SHOULDER BOX	60 seconds	15	2
FLAT-BENCH REVERSE FLY	60 seconds	14	3
LATERAL T-RAISE	60 seconds	12	2
JM PRESS	60 seconds	8	3
SINGLE-ARM TRICEPS CABLE PUSHDOWN	60 seconds	15	3
DIAMOND PUSHUP	60 seconds	12	3
HANGING KNEE RAISE	60 seconds	15	3
SIDE ISO AB	60 seconds	40 seconds	3

DAY 4

Exercise	Rest Interval	REPS	SETS
DEADLIFT	60 seconds	4	3
TRAP-BAR SHRUG	60 seconds	20	3
T-BAR ROW	60 seconds	8	3
DUMBBELL PULLOVER	60 seconds	12	2
FARMER'S WALK	60 seconds	20 yards	3
CHINUP	60 seconds	5	2
45-DEGREE BENT-OVER ROW	60 seconds	15	3
TIRE FLIP	60 seconds	10 yards	3
SIDE MEDICINE-BALL TOSS	60 seconds	12	3
DECLINE BENCH REVERSE CRUNCH	60 seconds	10	3

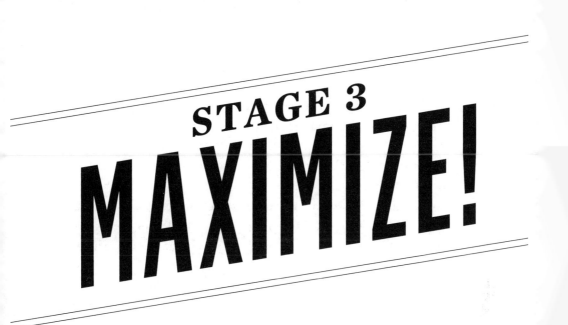

STAGE 3
MAXIMIZE!

Trimming your belly is the best route to more testosterone and massive muscle

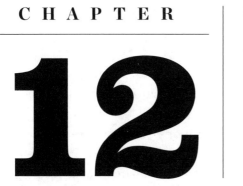

C H A P T E R

12

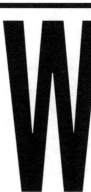

With just 4 weeks left to complete your testosterone transformation—and 8 weeks into the process—you're probably thinking, Hey, if

I get any more massive, I'll need new dress shirts! Well, there's more T where that muscle came from. The final 4 weeks ratchet up the intensity even further. "For this final stage, I want you to compete against yourself to maximize everything—the amount of testosterone you're trying to produce, the amount of body fat you're trying to burn off, the measure of strength you're trying to reach, and the amount of muscle hypertrophy you're hoping to see."

This stage features a new assortment of accessory exercises (core-stabilizing, multijoint, and isolation moves) to keep progressing, avoid injury, and ensure that your core muscles deliver the kind of power you'll need to move heavy loads. The volume of these Stage 3 exercises and strongman moves will remain high so you keep pushing your body to its limits. However, when it comes to your primary lifts—such as the deadlift, squat, and bench press—you will decrease the volume (reps and sets) but hoist more weight than in the previous stages. In addition, your rest between sets will become longer. More recovery time should allow you to achieve new maximum strength totals in each primary exercise, says Bryant.

Extra Tools For Extra T!

After completing Stages 1 and 2, you'll already have all of the unique tools that you'll need for Stage 3—an old tire and sledgehammer, a training sled, four 2x4 pieces of wood, and an old tractor tire. However, you'll need one more board in order to complete an exercise called the Five-Board Press.

Just as with the Three-Board Press, you'll use the extra boards to limit your range of motion even further when performing a bench-press movement, overloading your muscles at the point right before lockout.

The Stage 3 Workout

To begin Stage 3, perform a quick 5-minute warmup to loosen up your joints. Once you're warmed up, perform each exercise for the recommended reps and sets before moving on to the next exercise in the chart. (Again, if any exercise asks you to do between 1 and 8 repetitions, you'll prepare your muscles in the same way as described in Chapter 9.) Continue working your way through each exercise in the exact order presented in the chart, resting for the recommended number of seconds between each set.

HIGH-INTENSITY INTERVAL TRAINING MADE EVEN EASIER

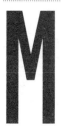

Maybe you can't spare 20 minutes for our HIIT workout. Maybe you find it too difficult or you don't want to bother timing 30-second intervals. That's okay. We have another option for you: a simple series of running drills that require no equipment except for a pair of running shoes and a stretch of flat surface on which to haul ass.

Sprint drills are a terrific companion to the TT strength program, because they take very little time and their explosive action builds leg strength, too. Have you ever seen the body of a world-class sprinter? Very different from a marathoner's body. These guys (and gals) own legs like tree trunks!

Find a place that allows you at least 25 yards of flat surface to run on. After you've warmed up properly (lightly jogging in place at a slow pace), you'll perform each sprint for the exact distance recommended. After each sprint, you can rest for up to one full minute—but no more than that.

HERE'S HOW YOUR 12-WEEK HIIT SPRINT PROGRAM BREAKS DOWN:

WEEKS 1 AND 2:
Sprint 20 yards (3 times), 40 yards (3 times), then finish by sprinting 60 yards (3 times).

WEEKS 3 AND 4:
Sprint 20 yards (twice), 40 yards (twice), 60 yards (twice), then finish by sprinting 80 yards (twice).

WEEKS 5 AND 6:
Sprint 20 yards (3 times), 40 yards (3 times), 60 yards (3 times), then finish by sprinting 80 yards (3 times).

WEEKS 7 AND 8:
Sprint 30 yards (twice), 50 yards (twice), 75 yards (twice), then finish by sprinting 100 yards (twice).

WEEKS 9 AND 10:
Sprint 30 yards (3 times), 50 yards (3 times), 75 yards (3 times), then finish by sprinting 100 yards (3 times).

WEEKS 11 AND 12:
Sprint 30 yards (twice), 50 yards (4 times), 75 yards (4 times), then finish by sprinting 100 yards (3 times).

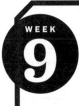

MAXIMIZE

DAY 1

Exercise	Rest Interval	REPS	SETS
BENCH PRESS	As needed	1	2
(FOR SET 1, TRY 90% OF YOUR 1RM; FOR SET 2, TRY ADDING A BIT MORE WEIGHT TO SET A NEW 1RM)			
BENCH PRESS	90 seconds	3	6
(FOR ALL SETS, TRY 80% OF YOUR 1RM)			
FIVE-BOARD PRESS	90 seconds	6, 4, 3	3
(SET 1, TRY 90% OF YOUR 1RM; SET 2, TRY 100% OF YOUR 1RM; SET 3, TRY ROUGHLY 10 PERCENT MORE THAN YOUR 1RM)			
REVERSE-GRIP BENCH PRESS	90 seconds	12	2
PARTIAL/FULL INCLINE PRESS	120 seconds	8	3
DUMBBELL CROSSOVER FLY	45 seconds	8	3
SCAPULAR RETRACTION	45 seconds	12	3
CHINUP	120 seconds	6	4
REVERSE FAT BAR CURL	90 seconds	12	4
SINGLE-ARM DUMBBELL SCOTT CURL	60 seconds	20, 15, 12, 20	4
BICEPS SLED CURL	60 seconds	60 yards	1
HANGING KNEE RAISE	45 seconds	15	3
ISO PRONE AB	45 seconds	60 seconds	3

DAY 2

Exercise	Rest Interval	REPS	SETS
SQUAT	As needed	3	2
(FOR SET 1, TRY 90% OF YOUR 1RM; FOR SET 2, TRY 95% OF YOUR 1RM)			
SQUAT	90 seconds	3	6
(FOR ALL SETS, TRY 80% OF YOUR 1RM)			
OLYMPIC PAUSE SQUAT	120 seconds	12	2
SINGLE-LEG ROMANIAN DEADLIFT	60 seconds	9	3
LATERAL LUNGE	60 seconds	12	2
GLUTE BRIDGE	60 seconds	10	4
STEPUPS	90 seconds	12, 10, 8	3
SINGLE-LEG GLUTE BRIDGE	30 seconds	12	3
MINI-BAND CLAMSHELL	30 seconds	10	3
STANDING PLATE TWIST	45 seconds	10	5
CALF RAISE	45 seconds	20	5
BARBELL COMPLEX	60 seconds	12	3
STANDING CABLE CRUNCH	45 seconds	12	3
BARBELL ROLLOUT	45 seconds	9	3

DAY 3

Exercise	Rest Interval	REPS	SETS
STANDING OVERHEAD PRESS	As needed	4	4
(FOR ALL SETS, TRY 90% OF YOUR 1RM)			
SEATED MILITARY PRESS (OVERLOAD)	As needed	4	3
OVERHEAD DUMBBELL FLY	45 seconds	15	3
SHOULDER BOX	60 seconds	12	3
FLAT-BENCH REVERSE FLY	45 seconds	15	3
SEATED LATERAL RAISE/LATERAL RAISE AND HOLD SUPERSET	90 seconds	12/30 seconds	4
DECLINE CLOSE-GRIP BENCH PRESS	90 seconds	10	4
PULLOVER TO PRESS (CLOSE-GRIP WITH EZ-CURL BAR)	90 seconds	15, 12, 8, 6, 20	5
DUMBBELL PAUSE FLOOR EXTENSION	45 seconds	15	3
HANGING LEG RAISE (STATIC HOLDS)	45 seconds	60 seconds	3
SIDE ISO AB	45 seconds	60 seconds	3

DAY 4

Exercise	Rest Interval	REPS	SETS
DEADLIFT	As needed	1	2
(FOR SET 1, TRY 100% OF YOUR 1RM; FOR SET 2, TRY ADDING 5% MORE WEIGHT TO YOUR 1RM)			
DEADLIFT	90 seconds	2	6
(FOR ALL SETS, TRY 80% OF YOUR 1RM)			
REVERSE SHRUG	90 seconds	15, 12, 10, 10, 40	5
BENT-OVER BARBELL ROW	90 seconds	15, 12, 6, 12	4
DUMBBELL PULLOVER	75 seconds	14	3
SINGLE-ARM LOW CABLE ROW	60 seconds	15	3
WEIGHTED CHINUP	150 seconds	4	4
45-DEGREE BENT-OVER ROW	60 seconds	15	5
SLEDGEHAMMER	90 seconds	Maximum	3
(MAXIMUM REPS EACH WAY FOR 60 SECONDS)			
TIRE FLIP	60 seconds	19 yards	5
OVERHEAD BARBELL SIDE BEND	45 seconds	12	3
LAND MINE	45 seconds	8	3

DAY 1

Exercise	Rest Interval	REPS	SETS
BENCH PRESS	As needed	1	2
(FOR SET 1, TRY 95% OF YOUR 1RM; FOR SET 2, TRY ADDING 5% MORE TO YOUR 1RM)			
BENCH PRESS	90 seconds	3	7
(FOR ALL SETS, TRY 75% OF YOUR 1RM)			
FIVE-BOARD PRESS	120 seconds	4, 3, 2	3
(SET 1, TRY 90% OF YOUR 1RM; SET 2, TRY 100% OF YOUR 1RM; SET 3, TRY ROUGHLY 10 PERCENT MORE THAN YOUR 1RM)			
REVERSE-GRIP BENCH PRESS	90 seconds	10	2
PARTIAL/FULL INCLINE PRESS	120 seconds	7	3
DUMBBELL CROSSOVER FLY	45 seconds	9	3
SCAPULAR RETRACTION	45 seconds	12	3
CHINUP	120 seconds	6	4
REVERSE FAT BAR CURL	90 seconds	13	4
SINGLE-ARM DUMBBELL SCOTT CURL	60 seconds	20, 15, 12, 20	4
BICEPS SLED CURL	60 seconds	70 yards	1
HANGING KNEE RAISE	45 seconds	15	3
ISO PRONE AB	45 seconds	60 seconds	3

DAY 2

Exercise	Rest Interval	REPS	SETS
SQUAT	As needed	2	2
(FOR SET 1, TRY 90% OF YOUR 1RM; FOR SET 2, TRY 100% OF YOUR 1RM)			
SQUAT	90 seconds	3	7
FOR ALL SETS, TRY 80% OF YOUR 1RM)			
OLYMPIC PAUSE SQUAT	120 seconds	10	2
SINGLE-LEG ROMANIAN DEADLIFT	60 seconds	10	3
LATERAL LUNGE	60 seconds	12	2
GLUTE BRIDGE	60 seconds	12	4
STEPUPS	90 seconds	12, 10, 8	3
SINGLE-LEG GLUTE BRIDGE	30 seconds	12	3
MINI-BAND CLAMSHELL	30 seconds	10	3
STANDING PLATE TWIST	45 seconds	10	5
CALF RAISE	45 seconds	20	5
BARBELL COMPLEX	60 seconds	11	3
STANDING CABLE CRUNCH	45 seconds	12	3
BARBELL ROLLOUT	45 seconds	9	3

DAY 3

Exercise	Rest Interval	REPS	SETS
STANDING OVERHEAD PRESS	As needed	3	4
(FOR ALL SETS, TRY 97% OF YOUR 1RM)			
SEATED MILITARY PRESS (OVERLOAD)	As needed	3	3
OVERHEAD DUMBBELL FLY	45 seconds	15	3
SHOULDER BOX	60 seconds	13	3
FLAT-BENCH REVERSE FLY	45 seconds	15	3
SEATED LATERAL RAISE/LATERAL RAISE AND HOLD SUPERSET	110 seconds	12/40 seconds	4
DECLINE CLOSE-GRIP BENCH	90 seconds	9	4
PULLOVER TO PRESS	90 seconds	15, 12, 10, 8, 15	5
DUMBBELL PAUSE FLOOR EXTENSION	45 seconds	15	3
HANGING LEG RAISE (STATIC HOLDS)	45 seconds	60 seconds	3
SIDE ISO AB	45 seconds	60 seconds	3

DAY 4

Exercise	Rest Interval	REPS	SETS
DEADLIFT	As needed	1	2
(FOR SET 1, TRY 100% OF YOUR 1RM; FOR SET 2, TRY ADDING 10% MORE TO YOUR 1RM)			
DEADLIFT	90 seconds	2	7
(FOR ALL SETS, TRY 84% OF YOUR 1RM)			
REVERSE SHRUG	90 seconds	15, 12, 10, 10, 45	5
BENT-OVER BARBELL ROW	90 seconds	12, 8, 6, 15	4
DUMBBELL PULLOVER	75 seconds	15	3
SINGLE-ARM LOW CABLE ROW	60 seconds	15	3
WEIGHTED CHINUP	150 seconds	5	4
45-DEGREE BENT-OVER ROW	60 seconds	15	5
SLEDGEHAMMER	100 seconds	Maximum	3
(MAXIMUM REPS EACH WAY FOR 65 SECONDS)			
TIRE FLIP	60 seconds	22 yards	5
OVERHEAD BARBELL SIDE BEND	45 seconds	12	3
LAND MINE	45 seconds	8	3

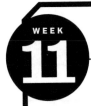

MAXIMIZE

DAY 1

Exercise	Rest Interval	REPS	SETS
BENCH PRESS	As needed	1	2
(FOR SET 1, TRY 95% OF YOUR 1RM; FOR SET 2, TRY ADDING 10% MORE WEIGHT TO YOUR 1RM)			
BENCH PRESS	90 seconds	3	8
(FOR ALL SETS, TRY 80% OF YOUR 1RM)			
FIVE-BOARD PRESS	120 seconds	3, 2, 1	3
(SET 1, TRY 90% OF YOUR 1RM; SET 2, TRY 100% OF YOUR 1RM; SET 3, TRY ROUGHLY 10 PERCENT MORE THAN YOUR 1RM)			
REVERSE-GRIP BENCH PRESS	90 seconds	8	2
PARTIAL/FULL INCLINE PRESS	120 seconds	6	3
DUMBBELL CROSSOVER FLY	45 seconds	10	3
SCAPULAR RETRACTION	45 seconds	12	3
CHINUP	120 seconds	5	4
REVERSE FAT BAR CURL	90 seconds	15	4
SINGLE-ARM DUMBBELL SCOTT CURL	60 seconds	20, 12, 8, 25	4
BICEPS SLED CURL	60 seconds	75 yards	1
HANGING KNEE RAISE	45 seconds	15	3
ISO PRONE AB	45 seconds	60 seconds	3

DAY 2

Exercise	Rest Interval	REPS	SETS
SQUAT	As needed	2	2
(FOR SET 1, TRY 95% OF YOUR 1RM; FOR SET 2, TRY ADDING 5% TO YOUR 1RM)			
SQUAT	90 seconds	3	7
(FOR ALL SETS, TRY 82% OF YOUR 1RM)			
OLYMPIC PAUSE SQUAT	120 seconds	10	2
SINGLE-LEG ROMANIAN DEADLIFT	60 seconds	10	3
LATERAL LUNGE	60 seconds	12	2
GLUTE BRIDGE	60 seconds	12	4
STEPUPS	90 seconds	12, 10, 8	3
SINGLE-LEG GLUTE BRIDGE	30 seconds	12	3
MINI-BAND CLAMSHELL	30 seconds	10	3
STANDING PLATE TWIST	45 seconds	10	5
CALF RAISE	45 seconds	20	5
BARBELL COMPLEX	60 seconds	11	3
STANDING CABLE CRUNCH	45 seconds	12	3
BARBELL ROLLOUT	45 seconds	9	3

DAY 3

Exercise	Rest Interval	REPS	SETS
STANDING OVERHEAD PRESS	As needed	3	3
(FOR ALL SETS, TRY 100% OF YOUR 1RM)			
SEATED MILITARY PRESS (OVERLOAD)	As needed	3	3
OVERHEAD DUMBBELL FLY	45 seconds	15	3
SHOULDER BOX	60 seconds	15	3
FLAT-BENCH REVERSE FLY	45 seconds	15	3
SEATED LATERAL RAISE/LATERAL RAISE AND HOLD SUPERSET	120 seconds	12/45 seconds	4
DECLINE CLOSE-GRIP BENCH	90 seconds	9	4
PULLOVER TO PRESS	90 seconds	15, 12, 10, 8, 15	5
DUMBBELL PAUSE FLOOR EXTENSION	45 seconds	15	3
HANGING LEG RAISE (STATIC HOLDS)	45 seconds	60 seconds	3
SIDE ISO AB	45 seconds	60 seconds	3

DAY 4

Exercise	Rest Interval	REPS	SETS
DEADLIFT	As needed	1	2
(FOR SET 1, TRY 100% OF YOUR 1RM; FOR SET 2, TRY ADDING 10% TO YOUR 1RM)			
DEADLIFT	90 seconds	2	8
(FOR ALL SETS, TRY 85% OF YOUR 1RM)			
REVERSE SHRUG	90 seconds	15, 12, 10, 10, 50	5
BENT-OVER BARBELL ROW	90 seconds	12, 8, 6, 15	4
DUMBBELL PULLOVER	75 seconds	15	3
SINGLE-ARM LOW CABLE ROW	60 seconds	15	3
WEIGHTED CHINUP	150 seconds	4	4
45-DEGREE BENT-OVER ROW	60 seconds	15	5
SLEDGEHAMMER	120 seconds	Maximum	3
(MAXIMUM REPS EACH WAY FOR 75 SECONDS)			
TIRE FLIP	60 seconds	25 yards	5
OVERHEAD BARBELL SIDE BEND	45 seconds	12	3
LAND MINE	45 seconds	8	3

MAXIMIZE

DAY 1

Exercise	Rest Interval	REPS	SETS
BENCH PRESS	60 seconds	5	3
REVERSE-GRIP BENCH PRESS	60 seconds	8	2
INCLINE PRESS	60 seconds	6	2
DUMBBELL CROSSOVER FLY	60 seconds	10	2
SCAPULAR RETRACTION	60 seconds	12	3
CHINUP	60 seconds	6	3
REVERSE FAT BAR CURL	60 seconds	15	2
SINGLE-ARM DUMBBELL SCOTT CURL	60 seconds	12	3
HANGING KNEE RAISE	60 seconds	15	3
ISO PRONE AB	60 seconds	60 seconds	3

DAY 2

Exercise	Rest Interval	REPS	SETS
SQUAT	60 seconds	5	2
OLYMPIC PAUSE SQUAT	60 seconds	6	2
SINGLE-LEG ROMANIAN DEADLIFT	60 seconds	10	2
LATERAL LUNGE	60 seconds	8	2
GLUTE BRIDGE	60 seconds	8	3
STEPUP	60 seconds	8	2
SINGLE-LEG GLUTE BRIDGE	60 seconds	12	3
MINI-BAND CLAMSHELL	60 seconds	10	3
STANDING PLATE TWIST	60 seconds	10	5
CALF RAISE	60 seconds	20	5
BARBELL COMPLEX	60 seconds	8	2
STANDING CABLE CRUNCH	60 seconds	12	3
BARBELL ROLLOUT	60 seconds	9	3

DAY 3

Exercise	Rest Interval	REPS	SETS
STANDING OVERHEAD PRESS	60 seconds	5	2
OVERHEAD DUMBBELL FLY	60 seconds	15	3
SHOULDER BOX	60 seconds	10	2
FLAT-BENCH REVERSE FLY	60 seconds	10	2
SEATED LATERAL RAISE	60 seconds	12	3
DECLINE CLOSE-GRIP BENCH	60 seconds	8	3
PULLOVER TO PRESS	60 seconds	12	3
DUMBBELL PAUSE FLOOR EXTENSION	60 seconds	12	3
HANGING LEG RAISE (STATIC HOLDS)	60 seconds	60 seconds	3
SIDE ISO AB	60 seconds	60 seconds	3

DAY 4

Exercise	Rest Interval	REPS	SETS
DEADLIFT	60 seconds	1	5
REVERSE SHRUG	60 seconds	15	3
BENT-OVER BARBELL ROW	60 seconds	8	3
DUMBBELL PULLOVER	60 seconds	15	3
SINGLE-ARM LOW CABLE ROW	60 seconds	10	3
CHINUP	60 seconds	6	3
45-DEGREE BENT-OVER ROW	60 seconds	15	3
TIRE FLIP	60 seconds	10 yards	5
OVERHEAD BARBELL SIDE BEND	60 seconds	12	3
LAND MINE	60 seconds	8	3

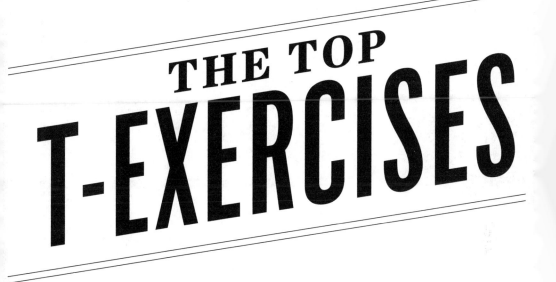

THE TOP T-EXERCISES

Detailed instructions for exercises in all three stages of the Testosterone Transformation Workout

C H A P T E R

13

T he exercises described in this chapter are listed alphabetically and according to the day in which they are scheduled, Day 1, 2, 3, or 4. Some moves are to be done on multiple days.

AB WHEEL HAND WALKING

MUSCLES TARGETED:
core, chest, shoulders, and triceps

THE
DAY 1
EXERCISES
FOR WEEKS 1 TO 12

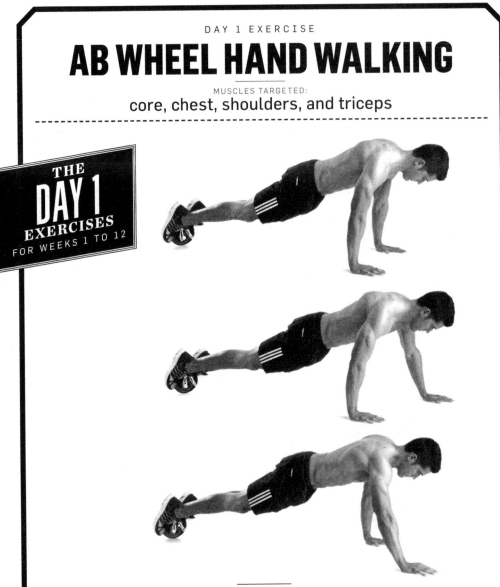

FOR THIS EXERCISE YOU'LL NEED AN AB WHEEL

START POSITION

➡ Place your hands flat on the floor (shoulder-width apart), keeping your arms straight, elbows locked. Straighten your legs behind you, keeping them together, and place the tops of your feet on the handles of an ab wheel.

THE MOVE: Pull in your stomach and contract your core muscles. Keeping your head in line with your torso, begin to walk forward with your hands, keeping your palms in line with your shoulders, for the required distance.

★ TRAINER'S TIP

Don't let your knees, head, or hips drop. Your body should stay straight from your head down to your heels in order to thoroughly train your core muscles throughout the movement.

BENCH PRESS

MUSCLES TARGETED:
chest, shoulders, and triceps

START POSITION

➔ Lie face up on an exercise bench with knees bent, feet flat on floor. Grab a barbell with an overhand grip, hands slightly wider than shoulder-width. Lift the bar off the rack and hold it directly above your chest, arms straight and perpendicular to the floor.

THE MOVE: Slowly lower the bar to your chest, then forcefully push the bar back up until your arms are straight, elbows unlocked. Repeat.

★ TRAINER'S TIP

Hold your breath as you lower the bar, and press it back up into the start position, taking a deep breath between each rep. Also, keep your head, back, and butt touching the bench at all times. Arching your back positions your body to allow other muscles—particularly your triceps—to help lift the weight, which removes effort from your chest while placing your lower back at risk of strain.

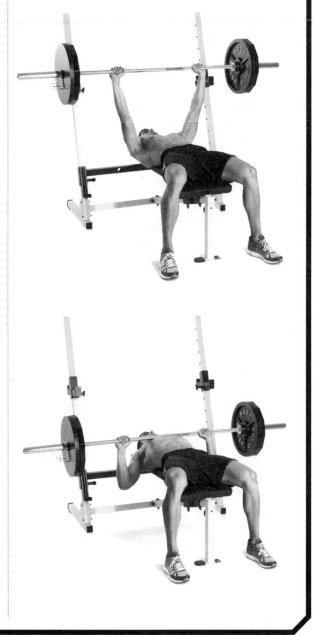

BICEPS SLED CURL

MUSCLES TARGETED:

posterior-chain muscle groups (quadriceps, hips, and core), plus upper back, biceps, forearms, and hands

START POSITION

➜ Attach a short bar to the training sled with a chain and grab it with an underhand grip. Stand facing the sled and step back until your arms are extended out in front of you at chest level, palms facing up. If it helps you, you can use a staggered stance, as shown.

THE MOVE: Bending your arms at the elbows, curl your fists to your sholders to drag the sled toward you. Once your fists reach your shoulders, take a step back with one foot so that you're in a split stance. As you step back, simultaneously let your arms extend in front of you so you can feel resistance from the bar. Continue the cycle—curl, then step backward—for the length of the exercise.

FOR THIS EXERCISE YOU'LL NEED A
TRAINING SLED

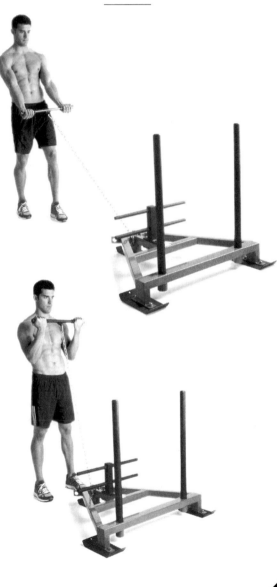

★ TRAINER'S TIP

Deciding how much weight to load onto the sled can be tricky for a newbie, but a good range to start with is about 50 to 100 pounds, depending on your size. After you perform your first set, you can either raise or lower the weight, depending on how the exercise feels to you. However, keep in mind that the type of surface on which you're pulling the sled will affect how much weight you can handle. For example, pulling the sled on a rubberized gym floor (with a towel under it to help it slide) will allow you to use more weight than if you try this exercise outside on grass or pavement.

BOTTOM END DRIVE

MUSCLES TARGETED:

chest, shoulders, and triceps

START POSITION

➜ Lie face up on an exercise bench with knees bent, feet flat on floor. Grab a barbell with an overhand grip, hands slightly more than shoulder-width apart. Lift the bar off the rack and hold it directly above your chest, arms straight and perpendicular to the floor.

THE MOVE: Lower the bar to your chest, then hold it there for 1 second. Forcefully push the bar back up, but only half the distance—you can have a training partner place his hand above your chest so you feel the bar touch it at the mid-point of the move. Immediately lower the weight back to your chest and repeat. After 5 partial reps, bring the bar back down to your chest for a final sixth rep, then push the bar over your chest until your arms are straight.

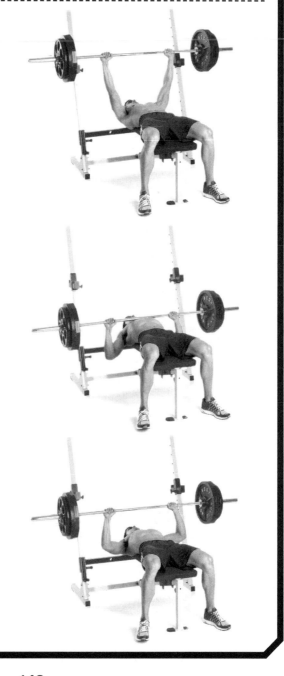

★ TRAINER'S TIP

This move helps to build power from the down position of the bench press, which is an area where many men tend to be weak.

CHEAT CURL

MUSCLES TARGETED:
biceps

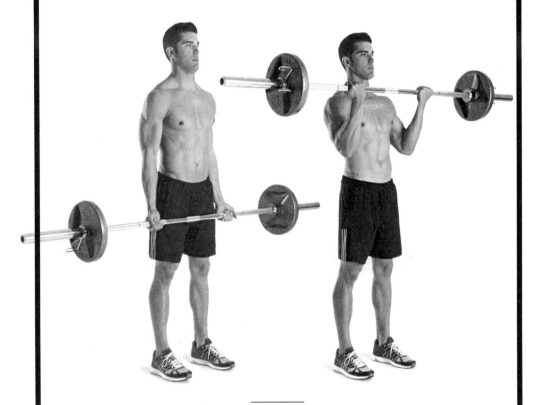

To do this exercise properly, load the barbell with 20 to 30 percent
more weight than you can usually handle for the required reps.
For example, if you're used to curling 100 pounds, load the bar with 120 or 130 pounds instead.

START POSITION

→ Stand holding the barbell with an underhand grip, hands shoulder-width apart.

THE MOVE: Quickly curl the weight up, using your hips and shoulders to help lift the load. Try to avoid raising your heels and coming up on your toes so that you don't lose your balance as you drive the weight upward. Pause at the top of the curl for 1 second, then slowly lower the weight for a count of 5 seconds. Repeat.

★ TRAINER'S TIP

Even if you're disciplined enough to pace yourself as you lower the weight, having a training partner place his palms right below the bar to prevent you from lowering the weight too fast can help you eke out better results.

CHINUP

MUSCLES TARGETED:

latissimus dorsi, rhomboids, lower trapezius, biceps, and forearms

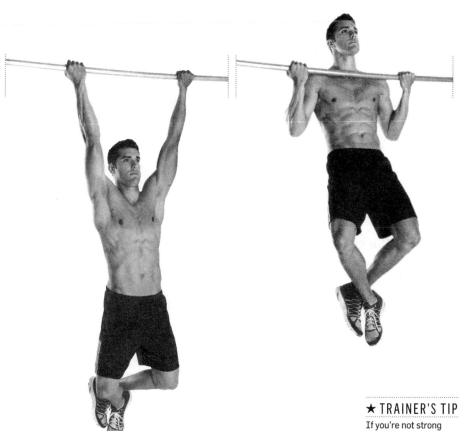

★ TRAINER'S TIP

If you're not strong enough to do this exercise for the required number of repetitions, attach one end of a stretch band to the chinup bar, let the other end hang down, then put one foot through the end of the band. This trick can help support a portion of your weight so that you're able to complete all the reps without sacrificing your form.

START POSITION

➜ Grab a chinup bar with a supinated grip (palms facing you), hands shoulder-width apart. Hang from the bar with your arms straight, elbows unlocked.

THE MOVE: Pull yourself up until your chin clears the bar. Lower yourself into the start position and repeat.

DUMBBELL CROSSOVER FLY

MUSCLES TARGETED:
chest

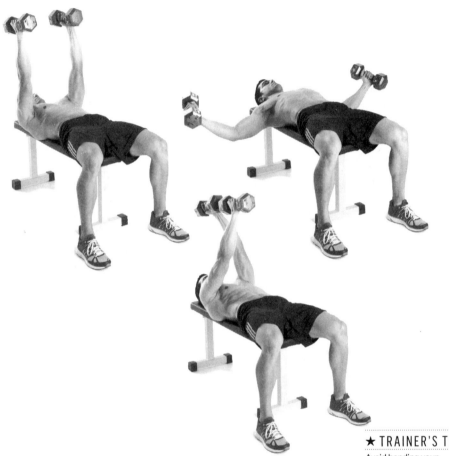

START POSITION

➜ With a light dumbbell in each hand, lie flat on a bench with your feet flat on the floor. Raise your arms above your chest, elbows slightly bent, with your palms facing each other.

THE MOVE: Keeping your arms in this position, sweep them down and out to your sides in an arc-like motion until the weights are at about chest level. Bring your arms back up, but instead of having the dumbbells touch at the top, cross your wrists over your chest instead—left hand over your right. That's 1 rep. Repeat the exercise once more, only this time, when you cross your wrists, do it so that your right hand crosses over your left. Continue to alternate wrist crosses.

★ TRAINER'S TIP

Avoid bending your elbows during the lowering and raising of the weights—a mistake that turns the exercise into more of a press than a fly and subsequently makes the move less difficult. Instead, bend your arms slightly before you perform the move, then keep your elbows locked in a bent position throughout the exercise.

FIVE-BOARD PRESS

MUSCLES TARGETED:
chest, shoulders, and triceps

START POSITION

➜ If you're an intermediate or advanced lifter, load a barbell with about 10 to 15 percent more than you would normally benchpress for the allotted rep range. Lie face up on an exercise bench with knees bent, feet flat on floor. Grab the barbell using an overhand grip, hands slightly more than shoulder-width apart, and start the exercise with your arms fully extended above your chest, your elbows in a locked position. Have your training partner place all five boards lengthwise on your torso (so that the boards run from your belly to the middle of your chest).

THE MOVE: Slowly lower the bar until it touches the top board, then explosively press the weight back up and repeat.

For this exercise, you'll need five small 2-by-6 pieces of wood and a training partner.

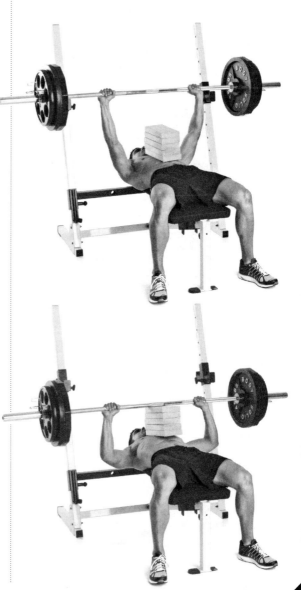

★ TRAINER'S TIP

If you don't have access to boards, you can also use a piece of Styrofoam or have a training partner place the flat of his palm at the same 10-inch height.

HANGING KNEE RAISE

MUSCLES TARGETED:
core and hip flexors

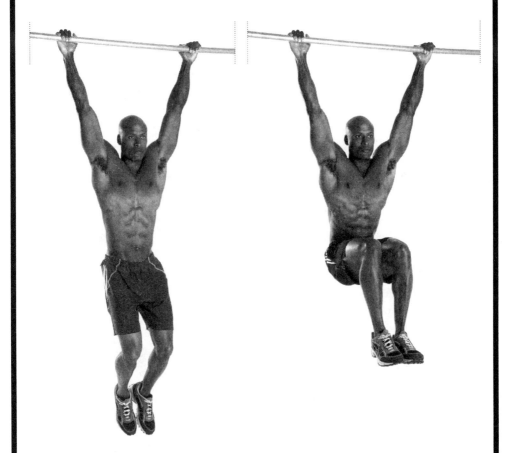

START POSITION

→ Hang from a chinup bar with your hands spaced more than shoulder-width apart. Your legs should be hanging underneath you, feet pointing to the floor.

THE MOVE: Bend and raise your knees until your thighs are parallel to the floor. Pause, then lower your legs. Repeat.

★ TRAINER'S TIP
Don't lift your pelvis and raise your knees simultaneously. Tilting your pelvis helps direct the stress of the move onto your abs instead of your lower back and hip flexors.

INCLINE DUMBBELL CURL

MUSCLES TARGETED:

biceps

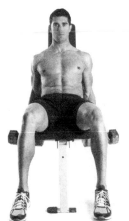
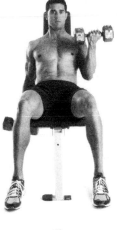
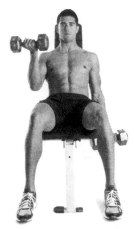
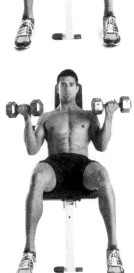

START POSITION

→ Lie back on an incline bench with a dumbbell in each hand. Your arms should hang straight down to the floor—so that they are angled behind your body, as opposed to in line with your torso—with your palms facing forward.

THE MOVE: Keeping your upper arms stationary, slowly curl the weight in your left hand only up to your shoulders. Lower the weight and repeat, this time curling just the weight in your right hand. Lower and repeat a final time, this time curling both weights up to your shoulders. That's 1 rep. Continue the pattern (left, right, and both) for the full set.

★ TRAINER'S TIP

Your back should stay glued to the back of the bench as you curl. Doing the exercise one arm at a time causes some men to "cheat" by leaning in toward the arm that is doing the curling. Leaving your torso on the bench keeps your upper arm where it needs to stay so that all of the effort is concentrated on your biceps.

INCLINE FLY

MUSCLES TARGETED:
chest

START POSITION

➜ Lie flat on an incline bench with a dumbbell in each hand. Raise your arms up above you so the weights come together directly above your chest. Your arms should have a slight bend in them, your palms facing each other.

THE MOVE: Keeping your arms fixed in a bent position, slowly sweep your arms down and out to the sides until the weights are in line with your chest. Sweep your arms back up to the start position above your chest, and repeat.

★ TRAINER'S TIP

Keep your arms slightly bent at the start of the exercise, but don't bend them at any point while performing the set. The goal of this exercise is to target only your chest muscles. By bending your elbows to lower the weights, you'll turn the move into a pressing exercise, which will allow your shoulders and triceps to assist your chest in lifting the weight.

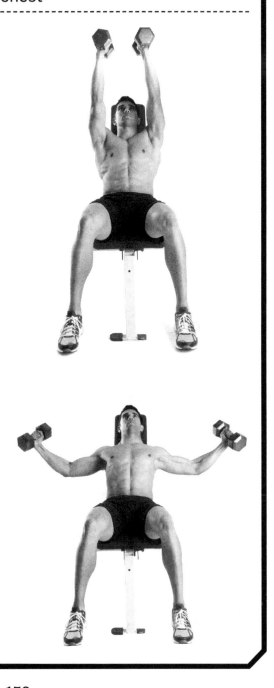

INCLINE FLY SUPERSET MAX PUSHUP

MUSCLES TARGETED:
chest, shoulders, and triceps

START POSITION

➡ Begin by performing one set of the Incline Fly (see previous page). Once you've completed one set, immediately pop off the bench and place your hands flat on the floor (shoulder-width apart), keeping your arms straight, elbows unlocked. Straighten your legs behind you, keeping your feet together, and position yourself so that the balls of your feet are touching the floor.

THE MOVE: Keeping your body in a straight line, bend your elbows and lower your chest to the floor. Push yourself back until your arms are straight (elbows locked), and repeat until failure.

This exercise combo requires you to do two exercises back to back with no rest in between.

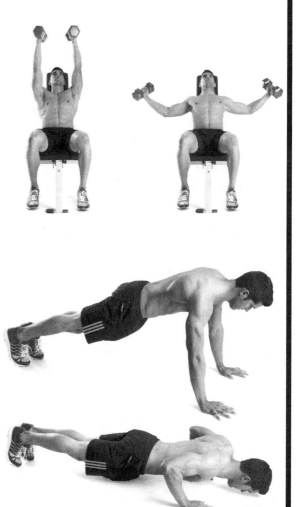

★ TRAINER'S TIP

You'll repeat the same two-exercise combination, doing both exercises back to back with no rest in between, for the remainder of the exercise. To get the best results, don't waste a single second in between. The entire object of this combo move is to exhaust your chest muscles before you start doing pushups, a tactic that will enable you to recruit even more muscle fibers than usual.

INCLINE I-Y-T

MUSCLES TARGETED:
all three muscle heads of the shoulders, plus the rotator cuff

START POSITION

➜ Set an incline bench at a 45-degree angle, then lie face down on the bench with your chest flat against the pad. Grab a light dumbbell in each hand and let your arms hang straight down from your shoulders—your hands should be turned so that your palms face each other.

THE MOVE: Keeping your arms straight (elbows unlocked), slowly raise them in front of you until your arms are parallel to the floor–the I position. Lower, then repeat, this time raising your arms at a 45-degree angle out from your sides—your body will look like the letter Y. Lower, then raise your arms once more, this time by extending them straight out from your sides (you'll look like the letter T). Lower, then repeat the entire three-move sequence for the duration of the exercise.

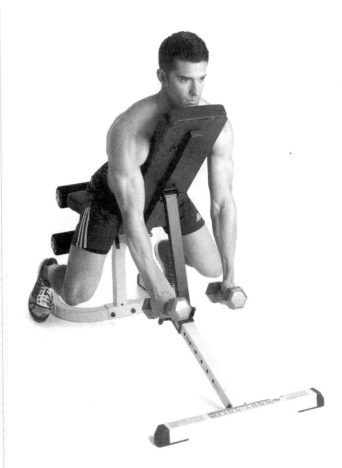

★ TRAINER'S TIP

Keep your head in line with your back at all times. Tilting your head back or turning to see your arms in motion will only increase your odds of straining your neck muscles.

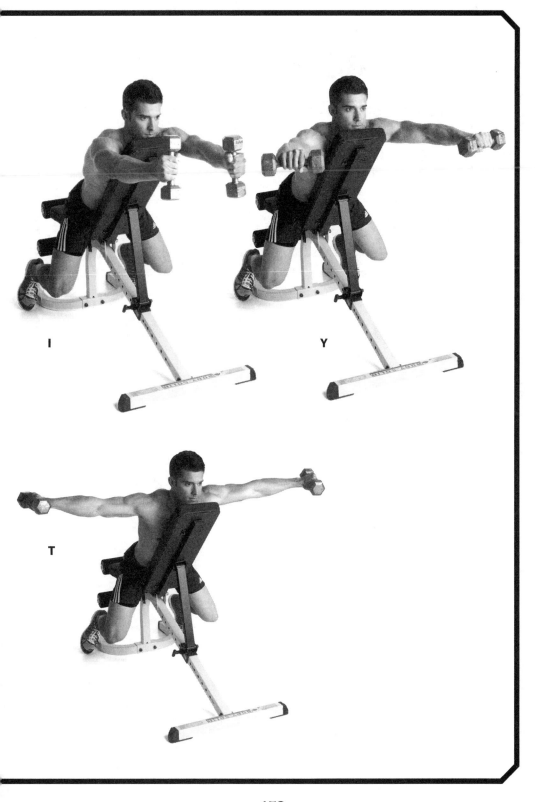

I

Y

T

INCLINE PRESS

MUSCLES TARGETED:

upper pectorals (plus shoulders and triceps)

START POSITION

➡ Lie back on an incline bench with your knees bent, feet flat on the floor. Reach up, grab the bar with your hands slightly more than shoulder-width apart, then lift the weight up so that the bar is directly over your chest. Your arms should be straight, elbows locked.

THE MOVE: Keeping your back flat on the bench and feet on the floor, inhale as you slowly lower the bar down to the top of your chest. Once it touches, exhale as you quickly press the bar back above your chest—elbows locked—and repeat.

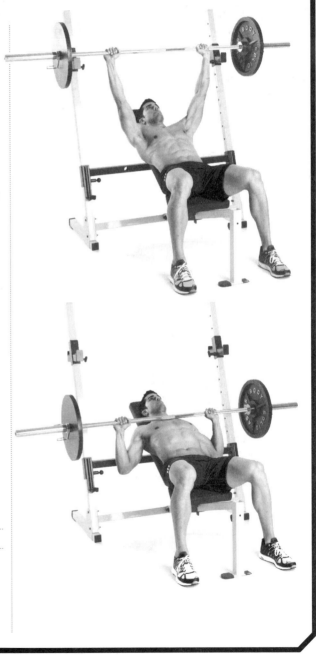

★ TRAINER'S TIP

To work your muscles through more angles—and see more development—just raise the bench one setting from the flat position for the first set. Keep raising the angle one setting every set afterwards, stopping once you reach a 35- to 40-degree angle.

ISO PRONE AB

MUSCLES TARGETED:
core

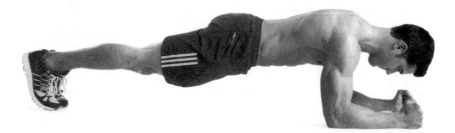

START POSITION

➔ Assume a pushup position with your legs extended behind you, your feet hip-width apart. Place your forearms flat on the floor so that your arms are bent at 90-degree angles. Your fists should point forward and your head should face down toward the floor.

THE MOVE: Keeping your head and back straight, contract your core muscles and hold this position for 60 seconds.

★ TRAINER'S TIP

Once the exercise becomes easier, try bringing your feet closer together. This trick challenges your balance even further, which will force your body to recruit more muscle fibers to stabilize yourself.

PARTIAL/FULL INCLINE PRESS

MUSCLES TARGETED:

chest, shoulders, and triceps

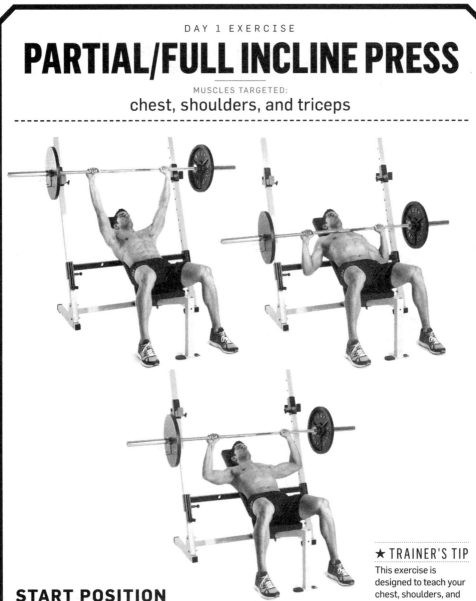

START POSITION

➜ Lie back on an incline bench with your feet flat on the floor and grab the bar with your hands slightly more than shoulder-width apart. Lift the weight off the rack and position it directly above your chest, arms straight and perpendicular to the floor.

THE MOVE: Lower the bar to your upper chest, then forcefully push the bar halfway back up. Immediately lower the bar to your upper chest once more, then repeat—raising the bar only halfway to lockout. Lower the bar again, then press the weight all the way up until your arms are straight, elbows locked. That equals one repetition. Continue this cycle—2 partial reps, 1 full rep—for the duration of the exercise.

★ TRAINER'S TIP

This exercise is designed to teach your chest, shoulders, and triceps to build more push-off strength at the bottom of the bench press, so don't push the bar up any higher than required. For best results, have a spotter place the flat of his hand above your chest at the midway point so you'll know when you've raised the bar to the right height.

REVERSE FAT BAR CURL

MUSCLES TARGETED:
biceps

START POSITION

➡ Stand straight, holding the bar with an overhand grip, hands shoulder-width apart. Your arms should hang straight down so that the bar rests in front of your thighs.

THE MOVE: Keeping your back straight and your elbows tucked into your sides, slowly curl the bar up to the front of your chest. Pause, lower the bar back in front of your legs, and repeat.

For this exercise, use a Fat Bar, Fat Gripz (www.elitefts.com), or wrap a pair of hand towels around the bar.

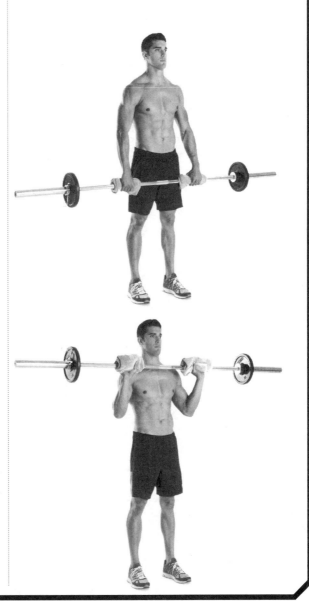

★ TRAINER'S TIP

Don't expect to lift as much weight as you normally can curl doing the exercise using a normal-width bar and a supinated grip (palms facing up). Try starting with a weight that's roughly 50 percent of what you would typically curl, then adjust accordingly.

REVERSE-GRIP BENCH PRESS

MUSCLES TARGETED:
upper chest, shoulders, and triceps

START POSITION

➡ Lie on a bench with your feet flat on the floor and grab the bar with an underhand grip, hands shoulder-width apart. Press the bar directly above your chest so that your arms are straight and perpendicular to the floor.

THE MOVE: Slowly lower the bar to your chest, then forcefully push it back up until your arms are straight, elbows locked. Repeat.

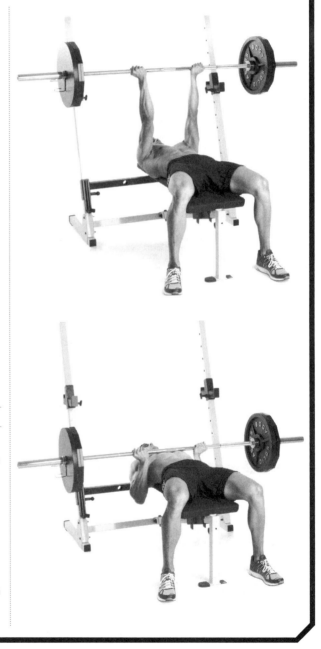

★ TRAINER'S TIP

This move will feel awkward at first, especially if you have a history of doing bench presses in the traditional way, so start light to get the feel. Also, grab a spotter when performing them, since it can be difficult to rerack the bar when using a reverse grip.

   If you don't have a spotter, try unracking the bar using a normal overhand grip, then lower it down to rest on your chest. Reverse your grip and perform the exercise as indicated. When you're ready to rerack it, lower it back to your chest, grab the bar with an overhand grip once again, press the weight back up, and rerack it.

SCAPULAR RETRACTION

MUSCLES TARGETED:

rhomboids and serratus

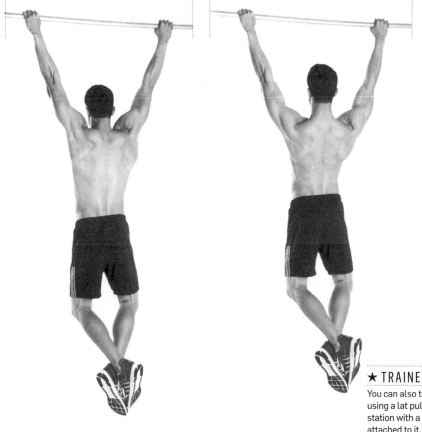

★ TRAINER'S TIP

You can also try these using a lat pull-down station with a long bar attached to it. Sit down at the machine, grab the bar with an overhand grip, and let your arms straighten out above you. Without bending your arms, draw your shoulder blades back as far as you can toward each other. Hold for a few seconds, return to the start position, and repeat.

START POSITION

➡ Hang from a chinup bar with an overhand grip, hands more than shoulder-width apart.

THE MOVE: Without bending your elbows, pull your shoulder blades down and back toward each other as far as possible. Hold this position for a few seconds, then return to the start position.

SEATED CABLE CURL

MUSCLES TARGETED:
biceps

START POSITION

➡ Place a preacher curl bench in front of a low cable pulley. Attach a small handle to the pulley, grab it with an underhand grip, then sit on the bench with your arms extended in front of you, upper arms resting on the pad.

THE MOVE: Moving only your forearms—any movement of your torso back and forth means you're cheating with your lower back— curl your fists toward your shoulders. Pause, lower, and repeat.

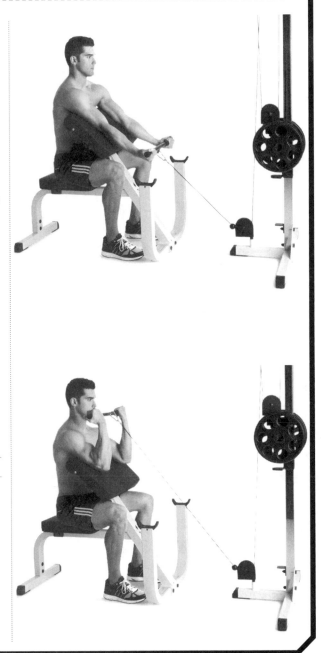

★ TRAINER'S TIP

Performing this type of curl during the routine is meant to give your body a break from the taxing curling movements you'll be performing for three straight weeks before.

If you don't have access to a cable station machine, you can also perform a basic standing dumbbell curl: Stand straight with a dumbbell in each hand, palms facing away from you. Bending your elbows, curl the weights up for a count of 2 seconds, then lower them for a count of 2 seconds.

SINGLE-ARM DUMBBELL SCOTT CURL

MUSCLES TARGETED:
biceps

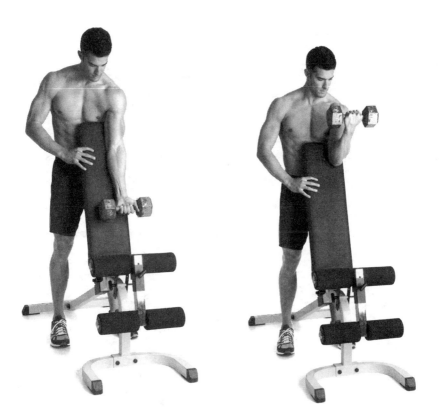

START POSITION

➜ Reverse the pad on a preacher-curl station so that the side your elbow leans against is perpendicular to the floor, or use the back of a leg extension machine, as shown. Lean over the pad, holding a dumbbell with an underhand grip, hands shoulder-width apart. Your arm should drape over the pad, pointing straight down to the floor.

THE MOVE: Keeping your upper arm against the pad, curl the dumbbell to your shoulder. Slowly lower the weight, and repeat.

★ TRAINER'S TIP

Your upper arm—from your armpit to your elbow—should remain flat on the pad at all times. Don't be afraid to lean over the pad to position your arm at the right angle if necessary.

SINGLE-ARM ECCENTRIC BARBELL CURL

MUSCLES TARGETED:
biceps

START POSITION

➜ Sit at a preacher-curl station and grab an Olympic-size barbell in the center of the bar with your left hand. Rest your upper arm on the slanted pad in front of you, palm facing up—the bar should already be in the up position of the curl, your left palm next to your shoulder.

THE MOVE: Slowly lower the bar for a count of 8 seconds, then pause for 1 second at the bottom. Have a training partner help curl the weight up to your shoulder or use your free hand to help you quickly bring the weight back up into the start position, then repeat.

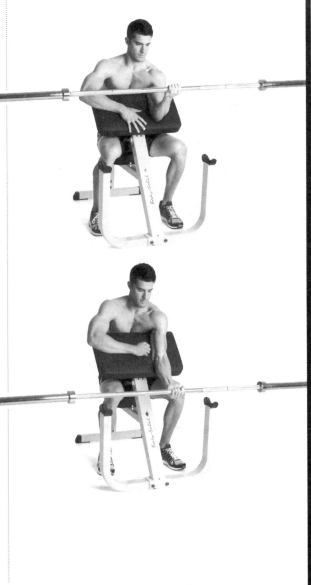

★ TRAINER'S TIP

Don't focus on your form or tempo as you curl the weight up. This exercise works your biceps through an eccentric contraction, so it's all about keeping your biceps muscles under tension on the down portion of the move.

SINGLE-ARM INCLINE DUMBBELL PRESS

MUSCLES TARGETED:
chest, shoulders, and triceps

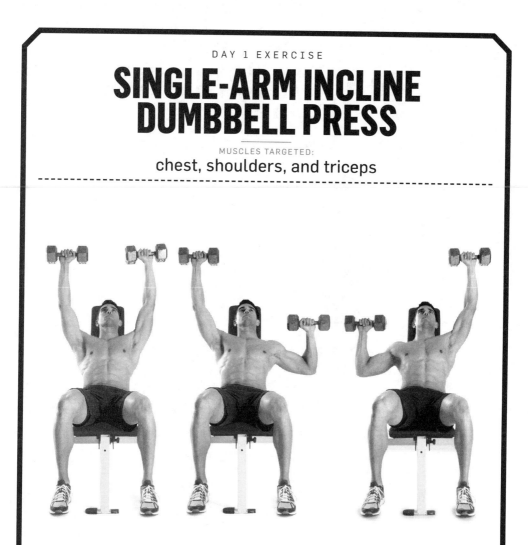

START POSITION

➜ Grab a pair of dumbbells and lie back on an incline bench with your legs bent and your feet flat on the floor. Press the dumbbells above your chest until your arms are straight, with your elbows in a locked position, palms facing forward.

THE MOVE: Keeping your right arm straight, bend your left elbow to lower the weight in your left hand down to the side of your chest. Press the dumbbell back into the start position, then repeat, this time lowering the weight in your right hand. Continue to alternate between your left and right arms for the duration of the exercise.

★ **TRAINER'S TIP**
Don't expect to lift the same amount of weight you could normally press. Because you're working each arm separately, you'll be doubling the time your muscles would be under tension when doing a normal set.

STANDING CABLE FLY

MUSCLES TARGETED:
chest

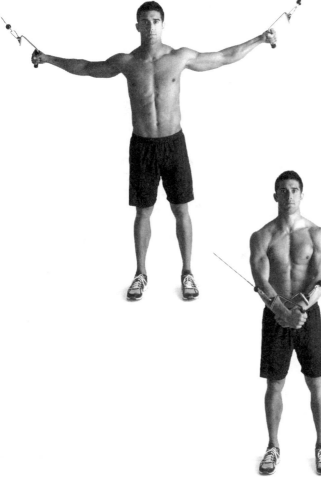

START POSITION

➜ Stand between two weight towers with your feet shoulder-width apart. Grab a high-cable handle in each hand—your arms should be extended straight out from your sides with your palms facing down. (You'll look like the letter T.)

THE MOVE: Keeping your arms straight and your elbows unlocked, slowly sweep them down in front of you, crossing your wrists just below your waist. Contract your chest muscles for 1 second, then slowly let your arms rise back up into the start position. Repeat.

★ TRAINER'S TIP

If you're a lighter guy, performing this exercise might pull you off-balance. If that's the case, try a staggered stance instead—one foot forward and one foot back, with your toes pointing straight ahead. This will give you more stability as you pull your arms forward. Just be sure you alternate which foot remains forward after each set to work your muscles evenly.

THREE-BOARD PRESS

MUSCLES TARGETED:
chest, shoulders, and triceps

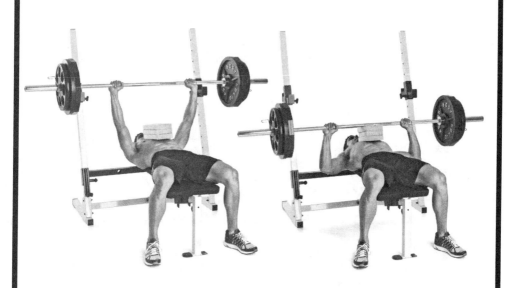

You'll need three short lengths of 2-by-6 lumber and a training partner.

START POSITION

➜ Load a barbell with about 5 percent more than you would normally bench press for the allotted rep range. Lie face up on an exercise bench with knees bent, feet flat on floor. Grab the barbell with an overhand grip, hands slightly more than shoulder-width apart, and start the exercise with your arms fully extended above your chest, elbows in a locked position. Have your training partner stack all three boards lengthwise on your torso so that the boards run from your belly to the middle of your chest.

THE MOVE: Slowly lower the bar until it touches the top board, then explosively press the weight back up and repeat.

★ TRAINER'S TIP

If you don't have access to boards, you can also use a piece of Styrofoam or have a training partner place his palm at the same 6-inch height as a guide.

ZOTTMAN CURL

MUSCLES TARGETED:
biceps

START POSITION

➜ Stand straight with a dumbbell in each hand, arms hanging straight down at your sides and palms facing forward.

THE MOVE: Keeping your upper arms stationary—and without rotating your wrists—curl the weights up until they're almost in front of your shoulders. At the top of the curl, gently rotate your wrists inward until your palms face forward. Lower your arms until they're just short of locking out, then finish by rotating your wrists outward until they once again face forward. Repeat.

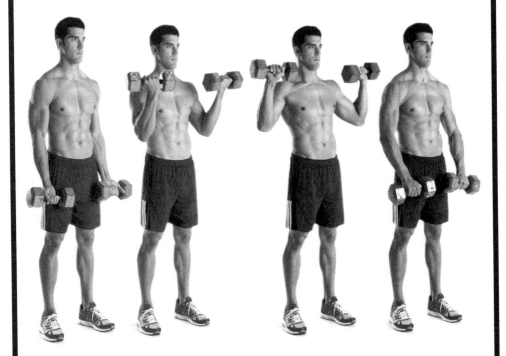

★ TRAINER'S TIP

The reason you need to stop just short of locking out your arms at the bottom of the move is to allow room to twist the weights without hitting your thighs. But don't think that your muscles are being robbed of results because you're not straightening your arms completely (which technically gives your biceps a split-second rest every repetition by removing the stress of the exercise). By never being allowed to straighten your arms, you are never relieving your muscles from their time under tension, so they are worked even harder as you go through the move.

ZOTTMAN CURL RACK-RUN

MUSCLES TARGETED:
biceps

START POSITION

➜ Stand holding a dumbbell in each hand, arms at your sides, palms facing forward.

THE MOVE: Curl the dumbbells up in front of your shoulders, pause, then rotate the dumbbells inward so that your palms face out in front of you. Lower the weights until your arms are just short of locking out, then rotate the weights outward so that your palms face forward once again (not shown). Do 8 reps, then choose a lighter pair of dumbbells that are roughly 20 percent lighter and repeat. Continue working down the rack, repeating the exercise using lighter weight each time, until failure.

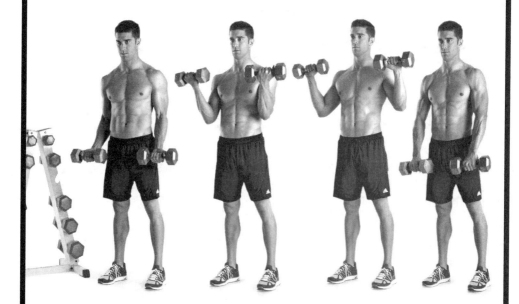

To do this exercise, you'll need a rack of various-size dumbbells that let you work your way down in weight. To start, choose a pair of dumbbells you can curl for 8 full repetitions.

★ TRAINER'S TIP

The point of this exercise is to thoroughly exhaust your biceps. It's critical to avoid moving your elbows too far forward. This shifts the effort from your biceps onto your front deltoids and wrist flexors.

BARBELL COMPLEX

MUSCLES TARGETED:
full body

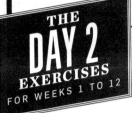

THE
DAY 2
EXERCISES
FOR WEEKS 1 TO 12

This exercise is actually a series of exercises that you'll perform one after the other with no rest in between to boost your anaerobic endurance and burn fat.

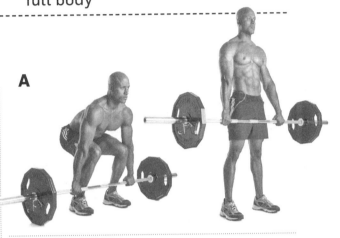

A

START POSITION

➡ Place an unloaded Olympic-size barbell on the floor and stand in front of it with your feet hip-width apart. Bend your knees and grasp the bar with an overhand grip, hands just beyond shoulder-width apart.

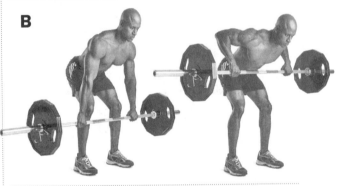

B

THE MOVE:

(A) DEADLIFT: With your chest up and back flat, quickly stand up—keeping the bar close to your body as you lift—until your legs are straight, knees unlocked. Quickly lower the bar to the floor and repeat for a total of 6 repetitions. Stop in the top position (bar against your thighs).

(B) BENT-OVER ROW: Bend at the waist and position your torso so it's nearly parallel to the floor, arms hanging straight below you. Quickly pull the bar up until it touches your midsection, then lower it. Do 6 repetitions, then stand up straight so that the bar rests along your thighs once more.

(C) CLEAN: Quickly shrug your shoulders as you pull the bar straight up. Your legs should

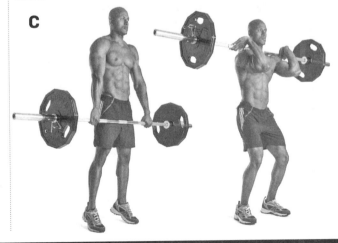

C

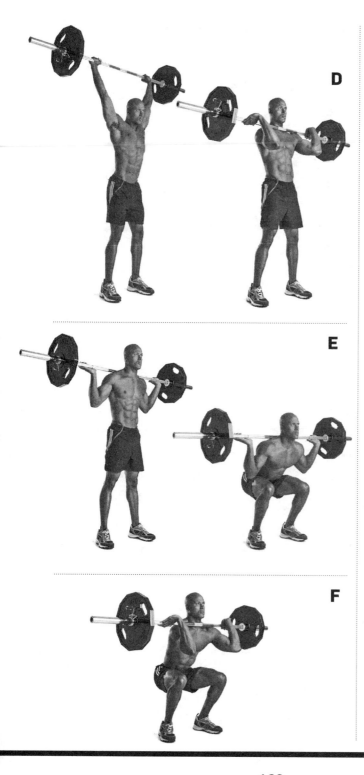

D

E

F

straighten as you rise up onto your toes. As the bar reaches your chest, bend your knees and swing your elbows forward to catch the bar on the front of your shoulders. Reverse the motion to return the bar down to your thighs and repeat for a total of 6 repetitions, stopping at the top position (bar in front of your chest).

(D) FRONT PRESS: Quickly press the bar up over your head, then quickly lower it back down to your chest. Do 6 repetitions, stopping at the top position (bar overhead).

(E) SQUAT: Lower the bar so that it rests on your upper back. Keeping your back flat, quickly squat down until your thighs are parallel to the floor, then quickly stand back up. Do 6 reps.

(F) FRONT SQUAT: Press the weight over your head, then lower it in front of you so that it rests across the upper part of your chest. Keeping the bar in place, quickly squat down until your thighs are parallel to the floor, then stand back up. Do 6 repetitions, then lower the bar back to the floor.

★ TRAINER'S TIP

The barbell complex is brutal but amazingly effective, so start light. It won't take long before you begin to add more weight to the bar. Just remember to do each repetition as fast as you can (without sacrificing form) and run through all 36 repetitions without resting or pausing in between.

BARBELL ROLLOUT

MUSCLES TARGETED:
rectus abdominis and core

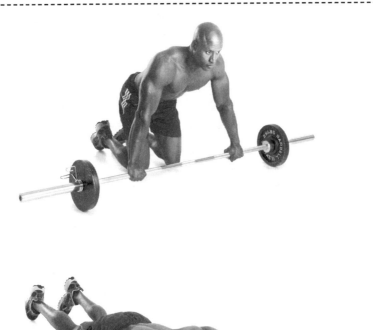

START POSITION

➡ Set a barbell on the floor, loaded with at least a 25-pound plate on each end. Kneel in front of the bar, then bend over and grab it with an overhand grip and your hands spaced just beyond shoulder-width apart. Only your knees and your toes should touch the floor.

THE MOVE: Keeping your knees on the floor, slowly roll the bar forward and away from you as far as you can. The goal is to roll the bar until your arms are almost in line with your body. Pause, then pull the bar back into the start position. Repeat.

★ TRAINER'S TIP
You can also use a 35- or 45-pound plate on either side. The bigger the plate size, the easier the move is to perform.

BODYWEIGHT LUNGE

MUSCLES TARGETED:
quadriceps, hamstrings, and glutes

START POSITION
➜ Stand straight with your feet hip-width apart and your hands at your sides.

THE MOVE: Take a big step forward with your left foot and lower your body until your left thigh is parallel to the floor. Your right leg should be extended behind you with only the ball of your right foot on the floor. Reverse the motion by pressing yourself back into the start position, then repeat the exercise by stepping forward with your right foot. Alternate between stepping forward with your left and right feet throughout the set.

★ TRAINER'S TIP
If stepping forward bothers your knees, try performing a reverse lunge instead. Again, stand with your feet together, then step back about 2 to 3 feet with your right foot. Bend your left knee and slowly lower yourself (your left knee should stay directly over your ankle). Stop before your right knee touches the floor, then push off with your right foot to get back into the start position. Repeat the move with your left leg.

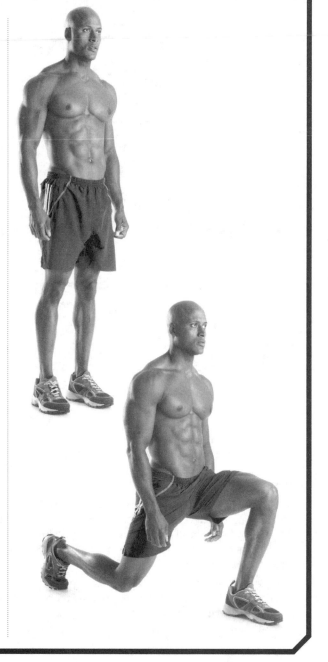

BULGARIAN ISOMETRIC SQUAT

MUSCLES TARGETED:
quadriceps, hamstrings, calves, and core

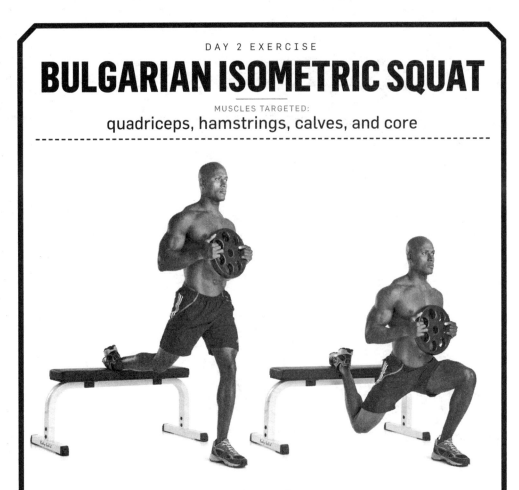

★ TRAINER'S TIP

This move isn't easy, so start with a light weight, or even your own body weight. If you're not using weight, place your hands on your hips throughout the move. (Extending them out in front of you or out to the sides makes the move easier, so you won't challenge your core muscles as effectively.) Eventually you can progress to resting a barbell across your upper back.

START POSITION

➔ Stand about 3 feet away from an exercise bench and turn so that your back is facing the bench. Grab a weight plate and hold it flat in front of your chest with both hands. Extend your right leg back behind you and rest your right foot on top of the bench—the top of your foot should be flat on the top of the bench.

THE MOVE: Bend your left knee and lower yourself until your left thigh is parallel to the floor. Hold this position for the required amount of time, then repeat the exercise, this time placing your left foot on the bench and bending your right knee.

CALF RAISE (on leg press)

MUSCLES TARGETED:
calves

START POSITION

➜ Sit in a leg-press machine with your back and butt flat against the back pad, feet spaced hip-width apart on the platform with the balls of your feet on the bottom of the platform (Your heels should hang off the platform.) Press the weight until your legs are straight, knees unlocked, then release the support bar.

THE MOVE: Without bending your legs, push the platform up as far as you can using just your toes. Pause for 1 second, lower the platform back to the start position, and repeat.

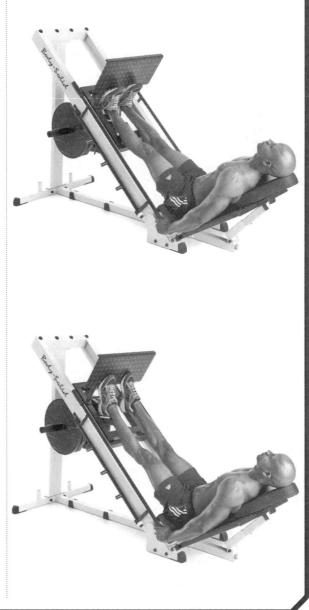

★ TRAINER'S TIP

If possible, take your shoes off—it increases your range of motion for more development.

FRONT SQUAT

MUSCLES TARGETED:

legs (primarily the quadriceps)

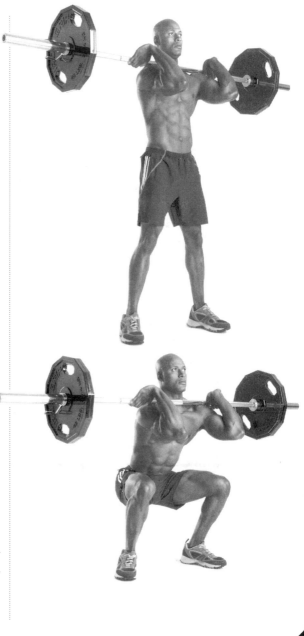

START POSITION

➔ Grab a barbell with an overhand grip slightly more than shoulder-width apart and rest the bar across the front of your shoulders. Raise your elbows in front of you so that your upper arms are parallel to the floor.

THE MOVE: Keeping your torso straight, slowly bend your knees and squat until your thighs are parallel to the floor. Push yourself back up until your legs are straight—knees unlocked—and repeat.

★ TRAINER'S TIP

Placing the bar in front of your body shifts more of the load off the hamstrings and gluteals and redirects it onto your quadriceps (thighs).

GLUTE BRIDGE

MUSCLES TARGETED:

glutes, lower back, core, and hamstrings

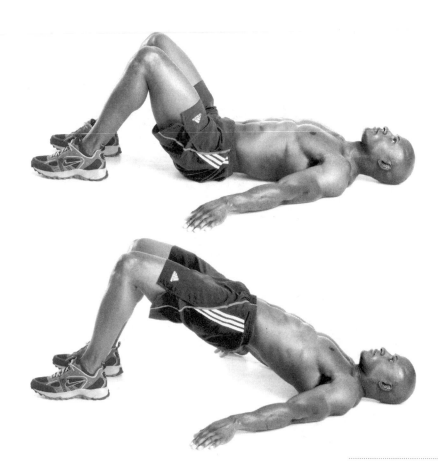

START POSITION

→ Lie on your back on a mat (or carpeted floor) with your knees bent and your feet flat on the floor. Extend your arms out from your sides for support.

THE MOVE: Pull your stomach muscles in, squeeze your glutes, then press down through your heels as you slowly lift your hips toward the ceiling. (Your butt, your waist, and, finally, your upper back should slowly rise off the floor.) Stop once your body forms a straight line from your knees down to your shoulders. Hold this position for 2 or 3 seconds, lower yourself to the floor, and then repeat.

★ TRAINER'S TIP

Don't push your hips too high. You won't get more results by raising them any farther than recommended—all you'll do is increase the risk of hyperextending your lower back. Keeping your abs tight throughout the exercise should prevent overarching.

HANGING WINDSHIELD WIPER

MUSCLES TARGETED:

transverse abdominis and obliques

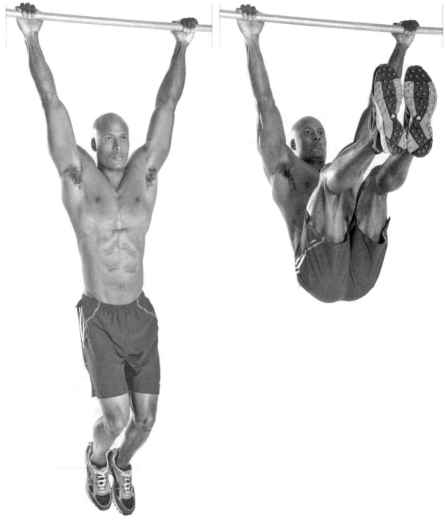

START POSITION

➡ Hang from a chinup bar with your hands spaced slightly more than shoulder-width apart. Your legs should hang straight underneath you, knees slightly bent with your feet pointing to the floor.

THE MOVE: Tilt your pelvis upward, then slowly raise your legs so your toes are roughly at the same level as your chest. Keeping your legs together and elevated, rotate them to the left so that your legs are parallel to the floor, then rotate them to the right. Continue to alternate back and forth, like a windshield wiper on a car, throughout the exercise.

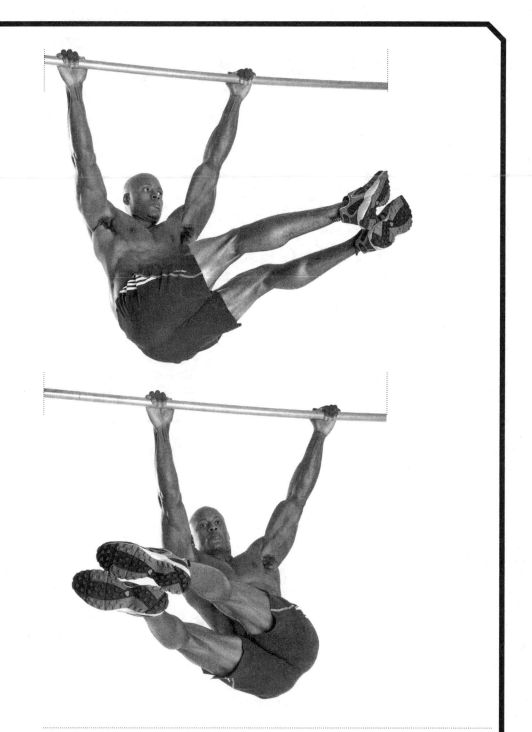

★ TRAINER'S TIP

Don't perform the exercise too quickly, since this can cause your muscles to waste energy decelerating your legs every time you swing them. Instead try to spend about 2 seconds rotating your legs from one side to the other.

TESTOSTERONE **177** TRANSFORMATION

HANGING LEG RAISE

MUSCLES TARGETED:
abdominals and core

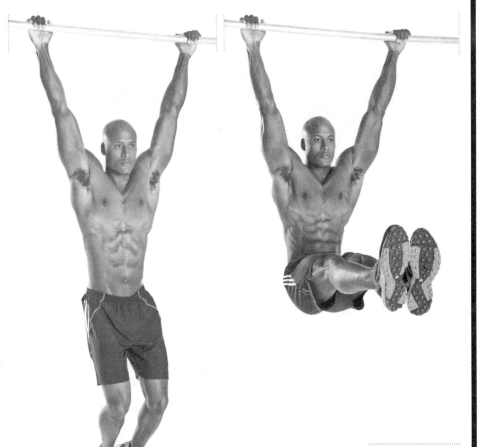

START POSITION

➡ Hang from a chinup bar with your hands spaced more than shoulder-width apart. Your legs should be slightly bent underneath you, your legs and feet together.

THE MOVE: Keeping your legs and feet together, raise your legs until they are parallel to the floor and your toes point toward the ceiling. Pause, then lower your legs back down.

★ TRAINER'S TIP

If you can't hold the move for 60 seconds, try it for as long as possible, take a 4- to 5-second rest, then go right back into position. Repeat until you reach 60 seconds—over time, you'll find you'll need fewer breaks and should be able to hold the posture for longer periods of time.

LAND MINE

MUSCLES TARGETED:
abdominals and core

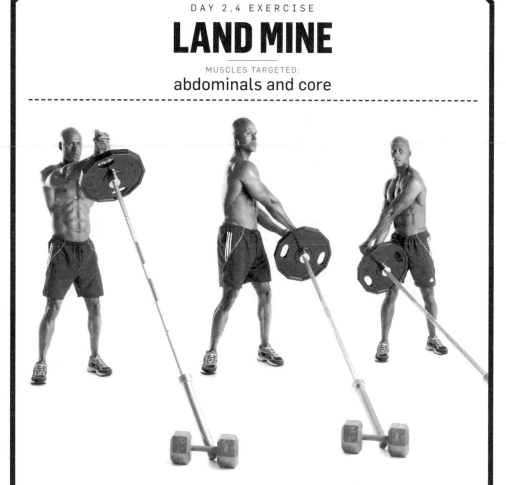

START POSITION

➡ Place one end of an Olympic barbell in the corner of the room or against a heavy dumbbell at an angle. Stand in front of the opposite end and grab it with both hands, one hand on top of the other. Position yourself so that your arms are straight in front of you, angled upward at about 45 degrees, with your feet hip-width apart. The opposite end should stay in the coner or touching the dumbbell to keep it from moving as you begin the exercise.

THE MOVE: Without moving your feet and while keeping your core muscles tight, twist to the left to lower the end of the bar across your body and down to your left side. Don't twist at the waist—this move is an anti-rotational exercise, so your core should stay tight and facing forward as you twist from the shoulders and upper back. Reverse the motion and twist to the right, lowering the end of the bar across your body and down to your right side. Continue twisting from left to right for the duration of the exercise.

★ TRAINER'S TIP

Once you become comfortable with this move, begin to add weight plates to the end that you're holding.

LATERAL LUNGE

MUSCLES TARGETED:

quadriceps, hamstrings, glutes, and adductors

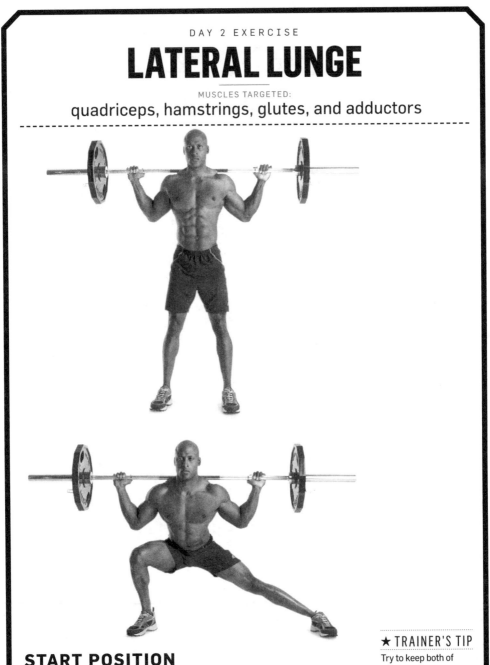

START POSITION

➥ Grab a barbell with an overhand grip and rest it along your upper back, then stand with your feet shoulder-width apart.

THE MOVE: Take a wide step out to the left and bend your right knee until your right thigh is parallel to the floor—your left leg will stay straight, with your foot planted on the floor. Push yourself back into the start position, then repeat the move by stepping to the right.

★ TRAINER'S TIP

Try to keep both of your feet pointing forward as you perform the exercise. Also, concentrate on pushing your hips backward as you lower your body into the lunge.

LEG CURL

hamstrings and glutes

START POSITION

➜ Lie facedown on a leg-curl machine, tucking your ankles under the pads. Your knees should hang just past the edge of the bench.

THE MOVE: Bend your knees and draw your feet toward your buttocks. Contract your glutes for 1 to 2 seconds, then lower your feet back until your legs are straight once more. Repeat.

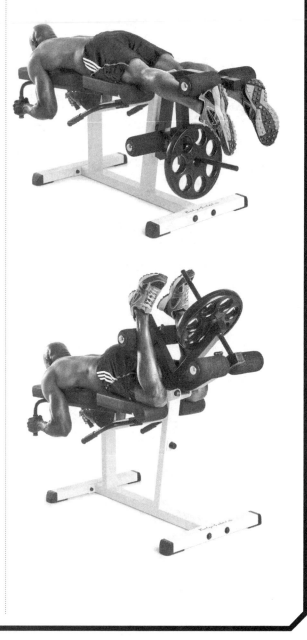

★ TRAINER'S TIP

If your chest lifts off the bench, you're probably using too much weight.

LEG EXTENSION

MUSCLES TARGETED:
quadriceps

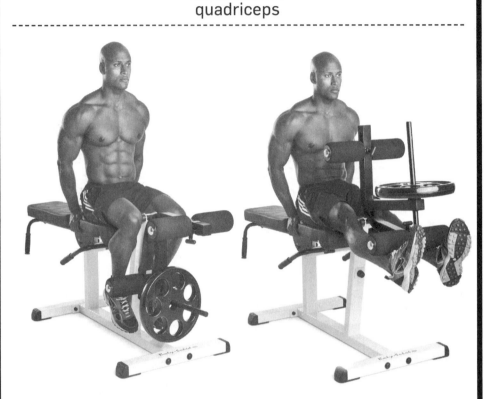

★ TRAINER'S TIP

Don't perform this isolation exercise too quickly or forcefully. Instead, focus on moving the weight in a slow and controlled fashion. Also, concentrate on resisting the weight as you lower your legs—don't let gravity do the work for you. The lowering phase of the lift is just as important as the raising part.

START POSITION

➜ Sit at a leg-extension machine with your ankles tucked under the footpads.

THE MOVE: Slowly extend your legs up and forward until they are both straight in front of you, knees unlocked. Pause, then slowly bend your knees until your legs are lowered back down.

MINI-BAND CLAMSHELL

MUSCLES TARGETED:
glutes and hip abductors

- -

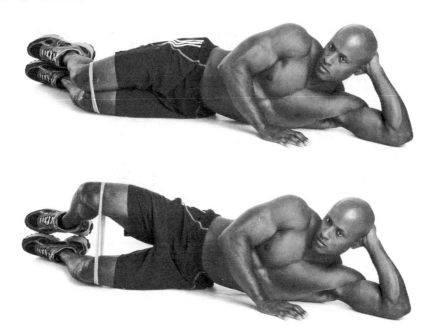

START POSITION

➜ Place your feet through a mini-band, then lie down on your left side with your legs and feet together, legs bent at 90 degrees. Pull the mini-band up until it's wrapped around your legs right above your knees. Bend your left arm and rest your head comfortably on your palm—your right hand can rest on the floor in front of you for support.

THE MOVE: Keeping your feet together, slowly raise your right knee as high as possible without rotating your pelvis. Lower and repeat for the required number of repetitions. When finished, switch sides to work the opposite leg.

★ TRAINER'S TIP

If you compare it with the rest of the exercises in this book, you might think this is the one to skip. Don't. This simple exercise might seem odd, but the move is designed to strengthen your external hip rotators, lessen lower-back pain, and prevent you from developing overuse injuries.

OLYMPIC PAUSE SQUAT

MUSCLES TARGETED:

quadriceps, hamstrings, and glutes

START POSITION

→ Place the bar on a squat rack about chest-high and stand in front of it. Grab the bar with an overhand grip slightly wider than shoulder-width, duck underneath it, and rest the bar across the back of your trapezius—not down along your shoulders. Lift the bar off the rack and step back from it.

THE MOVE: With your feet shoulder-width apart and your back straight, squat as deep as you can, then pause for 1 second. Press yourself into a standing position, knees unlocked, and repeat.

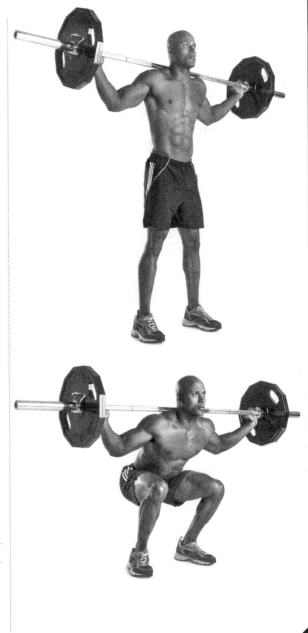

★ TRAINER'S TIP

This variation recruits a greater percentage of the muscle fibers within your quadriceps than are typically recruited by performing a regular squat.

SINGLE-LEG GLUTE BRIDGE

MUSCLES TARGETED:

glutes, lower back, core, and hamstrings

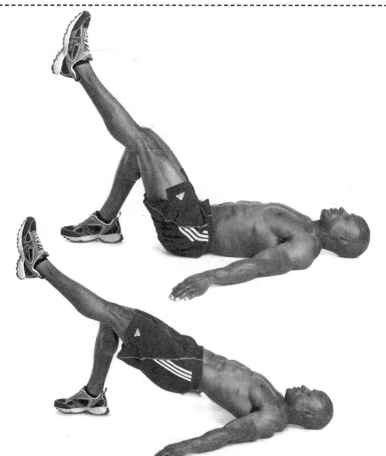

START POSITION

➜ Lie on your back on a mat with your knees bent and your feet flat on the floor. Extend your arms out from your sides for support. Raise and straighten your left leg so that it's at a 45-degree angle—your thighs should be in line with each other.

THE MOVE: Keeping your left leg extended, pull your stomach muscles in, squeeze your glutes, then press down through your right heel as you slowly lift your hips toward the ceiling. Your butt, waist, lower back, and middle back should rise off the floor. Stop once your body forms a straight line from your knees to your shoulders. Pause, lower to the floor, then repeat. After all reps, switch positions to work the opposite side.

★ TRAINER'S TIP

Never push off the ball of your foot—it makes the exercise less effective. Instead, make sure your foot stays flat on the floor or, to put more emphasis on your glutes, try raising your toes up so that only your heel touches the floor.

SINGLE-LEG PRESS

MUSCLES TARGETED:

quadriceps, hamstrings, glutes, and calves

START POSITION

➜ Sit in the leg-press machine with your back and butt flat against the pads and your right foot placed on the platform above you. Bend your left leg and rest your left foot on the floor in front of you and out of the way of the movement. Finally, press the platform up until your right leg is straight, knee unlocked, then release the support bar.

THE MOVE: Bend your right knee and lower the plate until your leg forms a 90-degree angle. Your foot should stay flat the entire time. Press the weight back up until your leg is straight (knee unlocked) and repeat. After performing the required number of repetitions, repeat the exercise with your left leg.

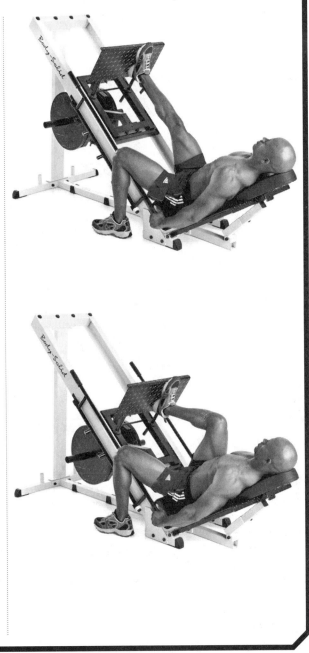

★ TRAINER'S TIP

Don't bend your legs farther than 90 degrees—you'll place unnecessary strain on your knees instead of focusing entirely on your leg muscles.

SINGLE-LEG ROMANIAN DEADLIFT

MUSCLES TARGETED:
hamstrings and glutes

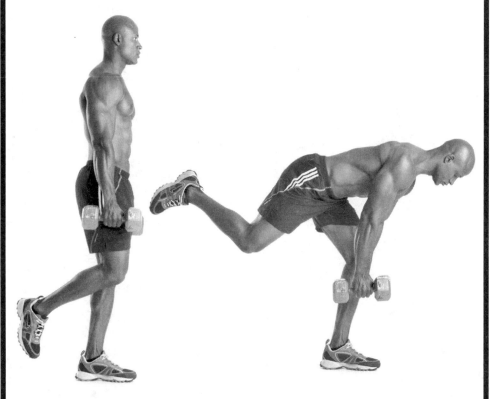

START POSITION

➜ Stand holding a dumbbell in each hand with your arms at your sides and your knees slightly bent. Lift your right foot behind you an inch or two off the floor.

THE MOVE: Maintaining this position, slowly push your butt backwards and lower your torso toward the floor as close to parallel as you can. (Your arms should hang straight down as you go.) Keep your lower back straight—don't round it as you bend forward. Hold for 1 or 2 seconds, then reverse the exercise by pushing your hips forward until you're back in the start position (still balancing on your left foot). Repeat for the required number of repetitions, then change positions to work the opposite leg.

★ TRAINER'S TIP
Keep the weights as close to your body as possible as you lower and raise them. This will focus all the effort onto your hamstrings instead of displacing it onto your lower back.

STANDING CABLE CRUNCH

MUSCLES TARGETED:
rectus abdominis (the 6-pack muscles)

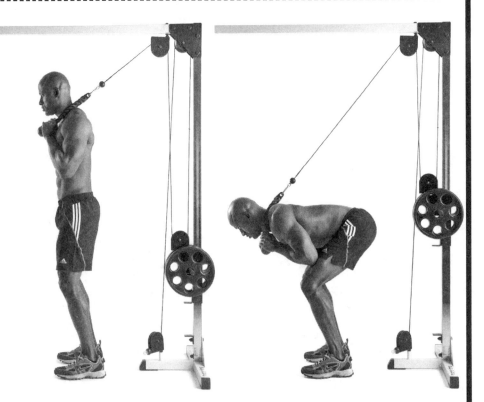

START POSITION

➜ Clip a rope handle to a high-cable pulley, grab an end in each hand, and stand with your back to it, knees slightly bent and feet shoulder-width apart. Place your fists down by your chest—elbows pointing down—so that the middle of the rope touches the back of your neck.

THE MOVE: Keeping your fists positioned by your chest, slowly bend forward at the waist until your elbows touch your thighs. Pause, slowly return to the start position, and repeat.

★ TRAINER'S TIP

Although this movement strengthens your midsection, it also helps open up your hips, which can allow you to perform some of the most effective T-building exercises, such as the deadlift and squat, more efficiently.

STANDING PLATE TWIST

MUSCLES TARGETED:
core

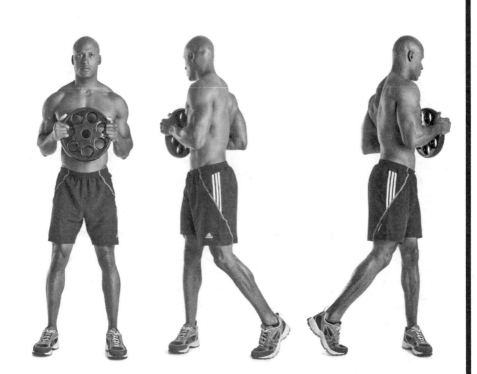

START POSITION

➜ Stand straight with your feet shoulder-width apart, holding a 25-pound weight plate in front of your chest. Bend your arms so that they're at 90-degree angles and tuck your upper arms into your sides.

THE MOVE: Keeping your upper arms locked in place, twist at the waist as far as you can to the right. As you go, raise your left heel off the floor and pivot off the ball of your left foot. Reverse the motion by twisting as far as you can to the left, this time raising your right heel and pivoting off the ball of your right foot. Continue alternating from right to left for the duration of the exercise.

★ TRAINER'S TIP

Don't stare straight ahead as you perform the move. Instead turn your head into each twist. Also, perform the motion at a normal pace—don't make the move explosive, which will only place your lower back at risk of injury.

STEPUP

MUSCLES TARGETED:

quadriceps, hamstrings, glutes, and calves

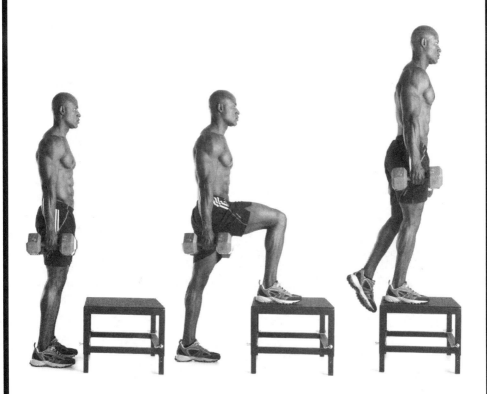

START POSITION

➜ Stand holding a dumbbell in each hand in front of a sturdy step. Let your arms hang at your sides (palms facing in toward your legs) with your feet about hip-width apart.

THE MOVE: Keeping your back straight, place your right foot onto the step. Push off with your left leg and stand up on the step so that you're balancing on your right leg only. Reverse the motion until you're back in a standing position in front of the step. Repeat the exercise—this time stepping forward with your left foot. Continue alternating between your right and left legs.

★ TRAINER'S TIP

If you like, you can use a staircase for this move instead of a bench. Just place your foot on either the second or third step, depending on your height and what feels more comfortable.

SQUAT

MUSCLES TARGETED:

quadriceps, hamstrings, and glutes

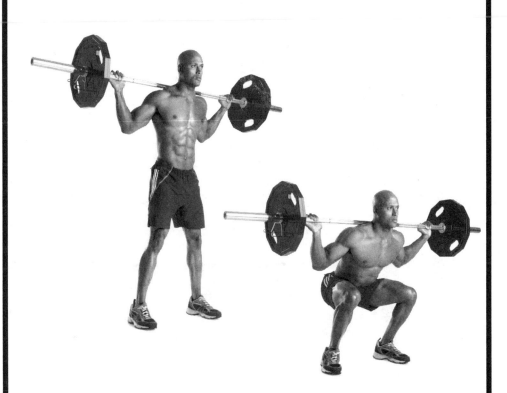

START POSITION

➜ Place the bar on a squat rack about chest-high and stand in front of it. Grab the bar with an overhand grip slightly more than shoulder-width apart, duck underneath it, and rest the bar across the back of your shoulders. Lift the bar off the rack and step back from it.

THE MOVE: With your feet slightly more than shoulder-width apart and your back straight, squat down until your thighs are parallel to the floor. Press yourself back up into a standing position, knees unlocked, and repeat.

★ TRAINER'S TIP

Focus straight ahead as you squat. Looking down at your feet while you squat can make you change the angle of the movement and make it harder to concentrate on staying balanced.

WALKING 45-DEGREE PLATE LUNGE

MUSCLES TARGETED:
quadriceps, hamstrings, glutes, calves, and core

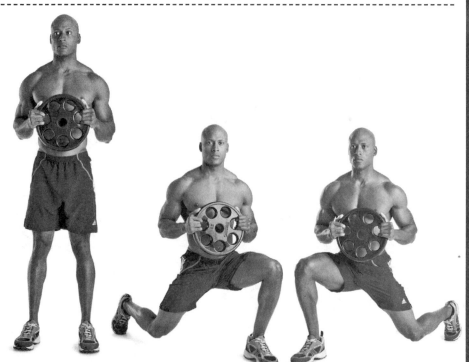

START POSITION
➜ Stand holding a 25-pound weight plate in front of your chest with both hands and your feet hip-width apart.

THE MOVE: Starting with your left foot, take a big step forward and to the side at approximately a 45-degree angle. Lower your body until your left thigh is parallel to the floor—your right leg should be extended behind you, with only the ball of your right foot on the floor. Next, step forward with your right foot, placing your foot out to the side at about a 45-degree angle. Lower your body until your right thigh is parallel to the floor—your left leg should be extended behind you, with only the ball of your left foot on the floor. That's one repetition. Repeat the cycle, alternating between your left and right legs, for the duration of the exercise.

★ TRAINER'S TIP

For this exercise, you'll need some space to walk forward. If you don't have enough room to work with, just take as many steps as you can, then turn around and do the exercise in the opposite direction—repeat as necessary.

ZERCHER SQUAT

MUSCLES TARGETED:
quadriceps, hamstrings, calves, core, biceps, and anterior deltoids

START POSITION

➜ Place a barbell on a squat rack at about chest height. Stand in front of the bar, place your arms underneath it, and rest the bar in the crooks of your arms—if you need to place a towel over the bar for cushioning, that's fine. Take the bar off the racks by taking a step back, then stand with your feet shoulder-width apart.

THE MOVE: Keeping your back straight as you go, squat down until your arms touch your thighs, then stand back up.

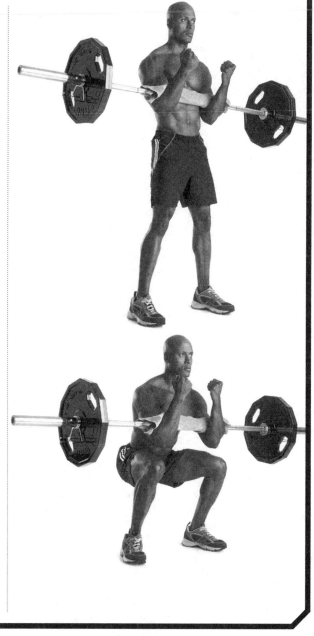

★ TRAINER'S TIP

This creative squat does two things that are unique among the many squat variations: It removes the element of pressure on the spine that's usually associated with squats, and it forces your core muscles to work even harder to keep your body stable as you go.

ARNOLD PRESS

MUSCLES TARGETED:

shoulders and triceps (plus upper trapezius)

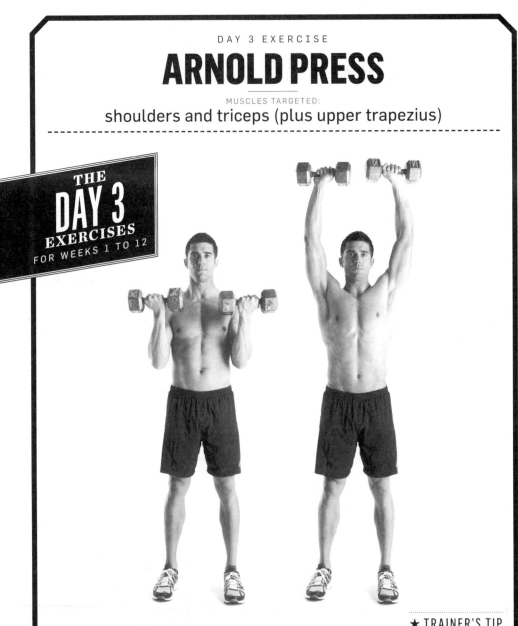

START POSITION

➜ Stand straight with a dumbbell in each hand. Bring the weights to shoulder height and close to the chest, palms facing in toward your body. Your elbows should be pointing down, your knuckles pointing toward the ceiling.

THE MOVE: Press the weights up over your head while simultaneously rotating your wrists outward. At the top of the movement, your palms should be facing forward. Lower the weights to your chest, rotating your wrists inward, until the weights return to the start position. Repeat.

★ TRAINER'S TIP

For some guys, performing this exercise takes a bit of coordination, so don't be discouraged if the move doesn't feel fluid at first. Eventually your muscles will begin to work in sync to make the exercise flow at a smoother pace.

CLOSE-GRIP BURNOUT

MUSCLES TARGETED:
triceps (plus chest and shoulders)

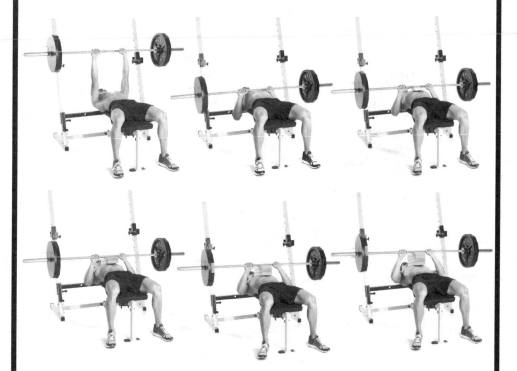

To do this exercise, you'll need four short lengths of 2-by-6 lumber and a training partner.

START POSITION

➜ Lie face up on an exercise bench with knees bent, feet flat on floor. Grab a barbell with an overhand grip, hands shoulder-width or less apart, and start the exercise with your arms fully extended above your chest and your elbows in a locked position.

THE MOVE: Slowly lower the bar until it touches the top of your chest, then quickly press the weight back up and repeat for 5 reps. Keeping the barbell pressed above you—don't rack it—have your training partner place one board lengthwise on your torso (so that the board runs from your belly to the middle of your chest.) Repeat the exercise for another 5 reps, lowering the bar down to the board. Continue to have your partner add one board every 5 reps to shorten the range of motion until you finish with four boards lengthwise on your chest.

★ **TRAINER'S TIP**

If you don't have access to 2-by-6s, you can also use 2-inch-thick pieces of Styrofoam. Or have a training partner place his palm 2 inches above your chest in lieu of a single board, then raise his hand 2 inches higher every 5 repetitions.

DECLINE CLOSE-GRIP BENCH PRESS

MUSCLES TARGETED:
chest, shoulders, and triceps

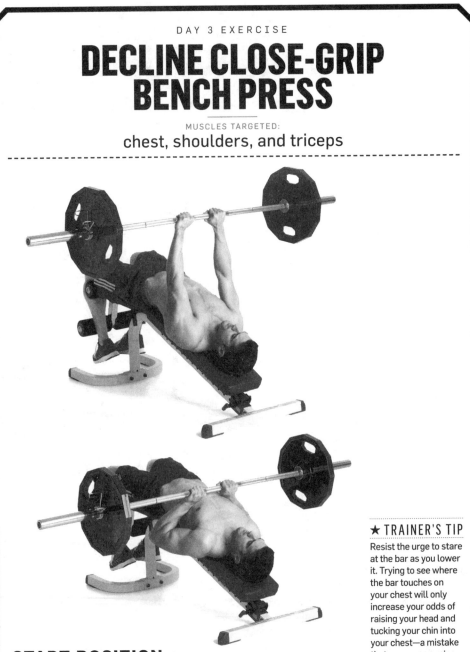

START POSITION

➜ Lie on a decline bench and have a partner hand you a barbell. Grab it with an overhand grip, your hands spaced slightly less than shoulder-width apart. Extend your arms so that the bar is directly above your chest, with your elbows in a locked position.

THE MOVE: Lower the bar until it touches your lower chest, then press the bar up until it's back in the start position. Repeat.

★ TRAINER'S TIP

Resist the urge to stare at the bar as you lower it. Trying to see where the bar touches on your chest will only increase your odds of raising your head and tucking your chin into your chest—a mistake that can compromise your breathing and increase your risk of straining your neck. Instead keep your eyes in line with your head and stare straight up as you drive through each repetition.

DECLINE CLOSE-GRIP BENCH PRESS (with EZ-curl bar)

MUSCLES TARGETED:
triceps

START POSITION

➡ Lie on a decline bench with your feet flat on the floor. Grab an EZ-curl bar with an overhand grip—hands spaced slightly less than shoulder-width apart—then press the weight directly above your chest. Your arms should be straight above you and your elbows in a locked position.

THE MOVE: Keeping your upper arms close to your sides, slowly lower the bar until it touches your lower chest. Press the weight back above you, keeping your elbows unlocked, and repeat.

For this exercise, you'll need an EZ-curl bar, which has a series of bends in it that help relieve stress on your wrists.

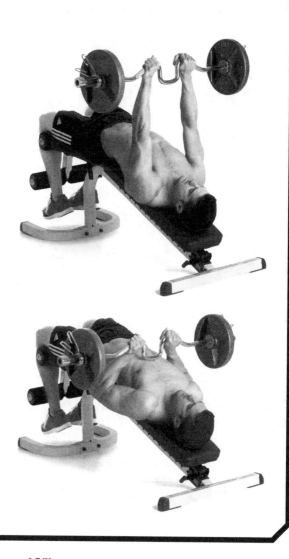

★ TRAINER'S TIP

Keeping your elbows unlocked at the top of the exercise keeps continuous tension on your triceps for the duration of the exercise. That's why resisting the urge to lock them at the top—which gives your triceps a break each time you do so—is the trick if you really want to exhaust your muscles thoroughly.

DIAMOND PUSHUP

MUSCLES TARGETED:

inner chest, shoulders, and triceps

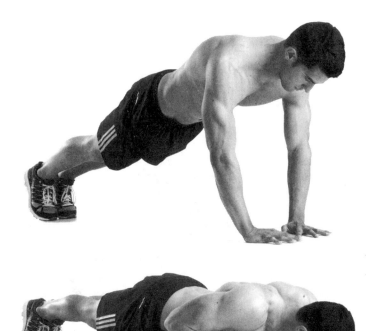

★ TRAINER'S TIP

Bringing your hands closer together involves more of your triceps than a regular pushup does. It also leaves you feeling off-balance, which recruits more proprioceptive fibers—a series of microscopic muscular nerves that explain to your brain where each part of you is at all times—so that the muscles throughout your arms, back, and legs instinctively react to help keep your body constantly balanced. The benefit: Your body will become faster at responding to upper-body imbalances, which can improve performance and prevent injuries.

START POSITION

➜ Place your hands flat on the floor with your arms straight, elbows locked. Position your hands closer together so that your thumbs touch, as well as your pointer fingers—the space between them should form a diamond shape. Finally, straighten your legs behind you, feet together, and position yourself so that the balls of your feet are touching the floor.

THE MOVE: Maintaining your balance, lower your body until your chest touches your hands. Pause, then push up, and repeat.

DUMBBELL PAUSE FLOOR EXTENSION

MUSCLES TARGETED:
triceps

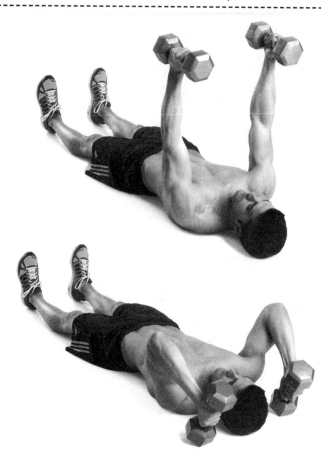

START POSITION

➔ Lie flat on the floor, holding a light dumbbell in each hand. Extend your arms straight up above your shoulders, palms facing each other.

THE MOVE: Keeping your upper arms stationary, slowly bend your elbows and lower the weights until the ends of the dumbbells touch the floor behind you. Pause for 1 second, straighten your arms up into the start position and repeat.

★ TRAINER'S TIP

By performing this exercise on the floor, you're limiting your range of motion, since the floor will naturally prevent you from lowering the weight farther down. This should allow you to use more weight than you would lift performing the same exercise on a weight bench.

FLAT-BENCH REVERSE FLY

MUSCLES TARGETED:
rear deltoids (plus upper and middle back)

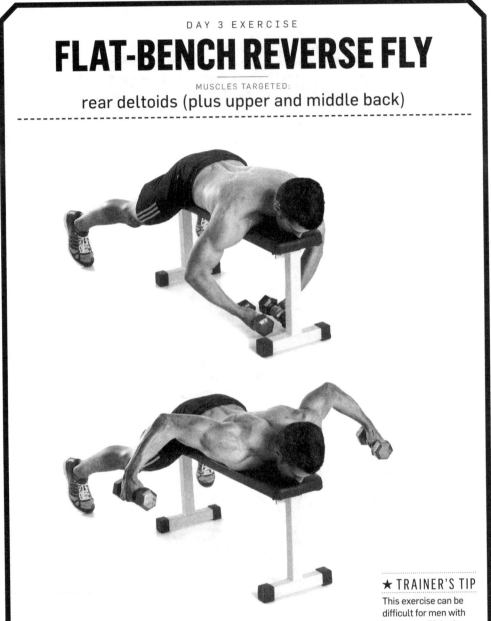

★ TRAINER'S TIP
This exercise can be difficult for men with long arms. If that's you, try starting the exercise with your arms bent even farther (up to just shy of a 90-degree angle) and/or try raising the bench by placing a sturdy exercise step underneath each end of the bench.

START POSITION
➜ Lie facedown on a flat bench with a light dumbbell in each hand. Let your arms hang down below you, palms facing each other, elbows slightly bent.

THE MOVE: Without raising your upper body off the bench, slowly raise the dumbbells up and out to your sides as high as you comfortably can. Pause, lower your arms, and repeat.

HANGING LEG RAISE (static holds)

MUSCLES TARGETED:
abdominals and core

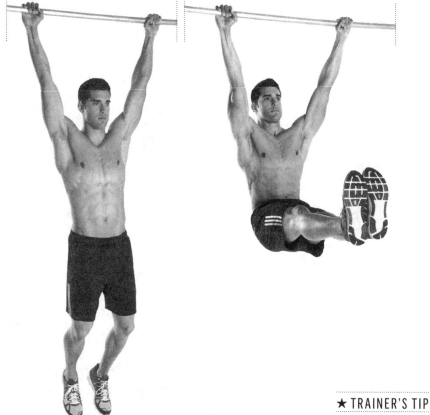

START POSITION

➜ Hang from a chinup bar with your hands spaced more than shoulder-width apart. Your legs should be slightly bent underneath you, your legs and feet together.

THE MOVE: Keeping your legs and feet together, raise your legs until they are parallel to the floor. Hold this position for 60 seconds, then lower your legs.

★ TRAINER'S TIP

If you can't hold the move for 60 seconds, hold for as long as possible, take a 4- to-5-second rest, then go right back into position. Repeat until you reach 60 seconds—over time, you'll find you need fewer breaks and should be able to hold the posture for longer periods of time.

JM PRESS

MUSCLES TARGETED:
triceps

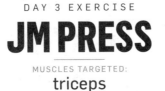

START POSITION

➜ Lie face up on an exercise bench with knees bent, feet flat on floor. Grab a barbell with an overhand grip, hands shoulder-width apart, and press it above you so that your arms are fully extended, elbows in a locked position. Instead of having the bar directly over your chest, line the bar up with your chin.

THE MOVE: Lower the bar toward your chin by bending your elbows. The bar should travel in a straight line up and down as you go, so let your elbows drift slightly toward your feet in order to allow the bar to stay on a straight path toward your chin. Once you bring the bar down as far as you can, reverse the motion by straightening your arms until the weight is back in the start position. Repeat.

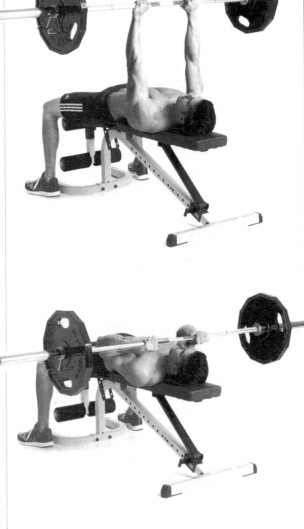

★ TRAINER'S TIP

If the bar drifts backward toward the top of your head, you're not letting your elbows naturally move forward as you lower the weight.

LATERAL RAISE

MUSCLES TARGETED:

medial deltoids (the sides of your shoulders)

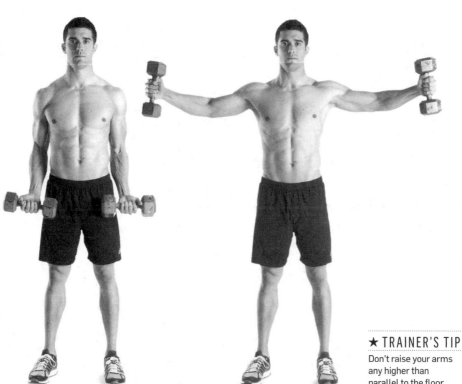

★ TRAINER'S TIP

Don't raise your arms any higher than parallel to the floor. Also, do not make the mistake of rotating your shoulders forward (as if you're pouring out two glasses of water).

Some men believe that this trick helps improve the effectiveness of the exercise, but all it does is boost your risk of developing shoulder impingement.

START POSITION

➜ Stand straight with your feet shoulder-width apart and a light dumbbell in each hand. Let your arms hang down at your sides, keeping a slight bend in your elbows, your palms facing forward.

THE MOVE: Keeping your elbows slightly bent, slowly raise your arms up and out from your sides until they are parallel to the floor—your body should resemble the letter T. Pause, slowly lower your arms to your side, and repeat.

LATERAL RAISE SUPERSET

MUSCLES TARGETED:
medial deltoids

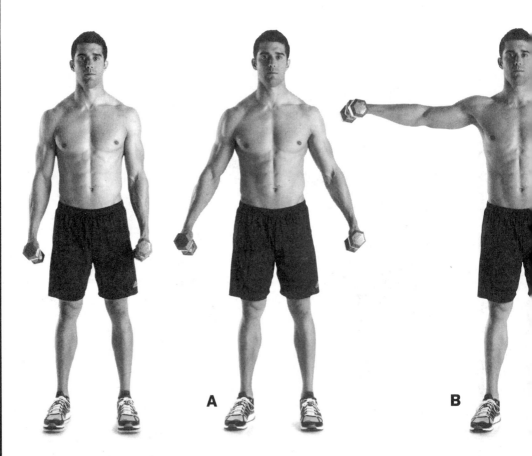

A

B

START POSITION
→ Stand straight with your feet shoulder-width apart and a light dumbbell in each hand. Let your arms hang down at your sides with your palms facing in.

THE MOVE:
(A) Raise your arms out to your sides until the weights are roughly 6 inches away from your legs, then lower them back into the start position. Do as many repetitions as you can in 20 seconds.
(B) Raise your arms out to your sides until your arms are parallel to the floor, then lower them back into the start position. Do as many repetitions as you can in 20 seconds.
(C) Bend your arms 90 degrees so that your forearms are parallel to the floor, palms facing in, knuckles pointing forward. Raise your elbows until your upper arms are parallel to the floor, then lower them. Do as many repetitions as you can in 20 seconds.

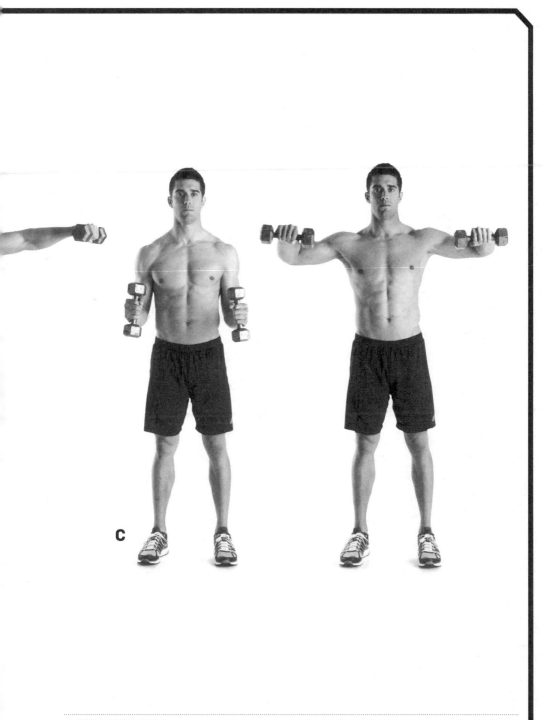

C

★ TRAINER'S TIP

Perform this exercise as rapidly as possible. Lift in front of a clock with a second hand, or have a friend time your 20-second segments with a watch.

TESTOSTERONE **205** TRANSFORMATION

DAY 3 EXERCISE

LATERAL RAISE AND HOLD

MUSCLES TARGETED:
medial deltoids

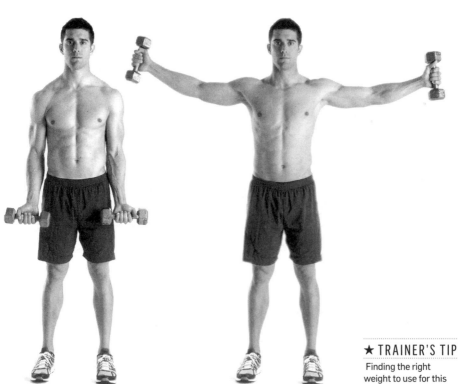

★ TRAINER'S TIP
Finding the right weight to use for this exercise can be tricky, but a good rule of thumb is to choose a pair of dumbbells you could raise out to the side for a total of 15 repetitions before exhausting your muscles. The ultimate goal is to use a weight that's challenging enough so that your muscles are screaming during the last 5 to 10 seconds of each set.

START POSITION
➜ Stand straight, holding a dumbbell in each hand, with your arms hanging down at your sides, palms facing forward.

THE MOVE: Without twisting your wrists, raise the weights up until your arms are parallel to the floor. Hold this position for the required amount of time, then lower your arms to your sides.

LATERAL T-RAISE

medial deltoids

START POSITION

➜ Stand straight with a dumbbell in each hand and your arms bent at 90-degree angles. Your forearms should be parallel to the floor with palms facing in, knuckles pointing forward.

THE MOVE: Maintaining this position, raise your elbows out to your sides until your palms are facing down toward the floor—your elbows and upper arms should form a straight line. Lower your arms to the start position and repeat.

★ TRAINER'S TIP

Keep your arms bent at 90-degree angles for the entire movement, but don't look down to make sure you're using proper form—this can place unnecessary stress on the muscles along your upper trapezius and throughout your neck.

Instead, try to do the exercise in front of a mirror so that you can keep your head in line with your back the entire time.

OVERHEAD DUMBBELL FLY

MUSCLES TARGETED:
medial deltoids

START POSITION

➜ Stand straight with a light dumbbell in each hand and your feet shoulder-width apart. Press the weights straight over your shoulders and turn your wrists so that your palms face each other—your arms should have a slight bend in them.

THE MOVE: Keeping your elbows fixed in a slightly bent position, slowly sweep your arms down and out from your sides until they are parallel to the floor. Your body should look like the letter T. Pause, then reverse the motion until your arms are in the start position. Repeat.

★ TRAINER'S TIP

If you feel any unusual discomfort in your shoulders—besides the obvious muscular pain you should be feeling as you exhaust them—try starting the exercise by twisting your wrists so that your palms face forward instead of toward each other. This should make the move a bit easier on your shoulder joints.

PAUL DICKS PRESS

MUSCLES TARGETED:
triceps

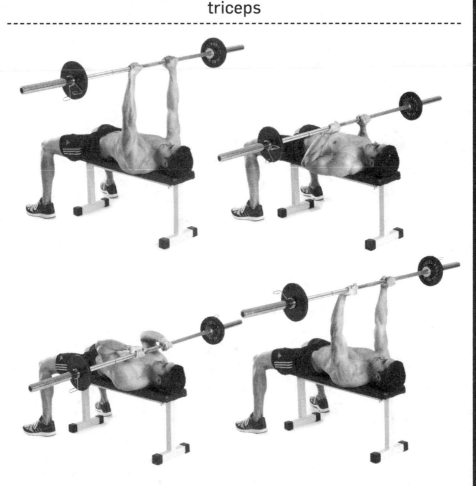

START POSITION

➜ Lie face up on an exercise bench with knees bent, feet flat on floor. Grab a barbell with an overhand grip, hands shoulder-width apart, then press it above your chest so that your arms are fully extended, elbows locked.

THE MOVE: Keeping your elbows in, lower the bar to your chest. Once the bar is lowered to about an inch from your chest, roll your elbows up as you shift the bar backward toward your chin. Maintaining this position, press the weight back up—leading with your fists—until your arms are straight once more. Repeat.

★ TRAINER'S TIP

This powerful exercise works like three triceps exercises simultaneously: a close-grip bench press, a triceps pressdown, and a skull crusher. Start with an empty bar. Add weight once you are accustomed to the exercise.

PULLOVER TO PRESS

MUSCLES TARGETED:

chest, back, shoulders, and triceps

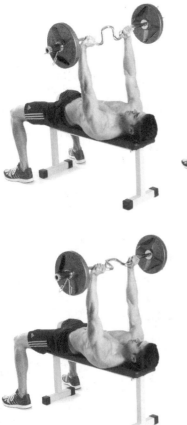
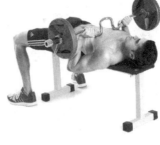

START POSITION

➡ Grab a loaded EZ-curl bar with an overhand grip, hands shoulder-width apart or closer. Lie back on a flat bench so that the top of your head is at the very end. Press the bar over your chest until your arms are straight, elbows unlocked.

THE MOVE: Keeping your elbows slightly bent, slowly lower the bar backward in an arc behind your head until your upper arms are in line with your head. Pause, then pull the weight back into the start position. Bend your elbows and lower the bar down to your chest. Press the bar back into the start position. That's one repetition. Repeat the two-part cycle (pullover/press) for the duration of the exercise.

★ TRAINER'S TIP

Here's a trick: If your pullovers tire out first because your back is exhausted, then try doing the pressing portion at a pace 1 or 2 seconds slower. If your presses tire out first because your chest muscles are weaker, do the pullover portion at a pace 1 or 2 seconds slower.

Tweaking the pace so that you spend more time contracting whichever muscle group is stronger should even things out so that both muscle groups become exhausted at the same time.

REAR-DELT FLY

MUSCLES TARGETED:
posterior deltoids (back of your shoulders)

START POSITION

➜ Stand straight with your knees slightly bent and a light dumbbell in each hand. Keeping your back flat, bend from the waist and lean forward until your torso is parallel to the floor. Let your arms hang straight down below you, palms facing each other.

THE MOVE: Slowly raise the dumbbells out to your sides until your arms are parallel to the floor. Pause, lower your arms, and repeat.

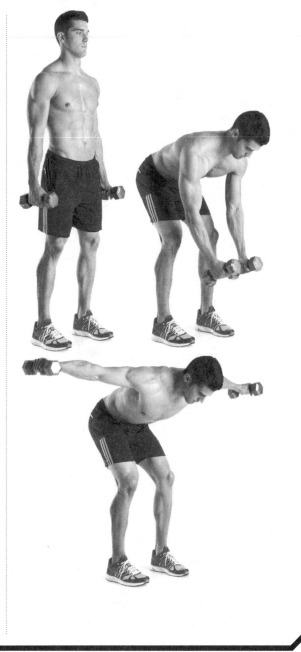

★ TRAINER'S TIP

Try not to lift your torso as you raise the weights—that means you're using momentum and your lower back to cheat the weights upward. Instead focus on making sure that only your arms are moving during the exercise.

SEATED LATERAL RAISE

MUSCLES TARGETED:
medial deltoids

START POSITION

→ Sit on an exercise bench with a light dumbbell in each hand and your feet flat on the floor. Your arms should hang straight down at your sides with your palms facing in toward each other.

THE MOVE: Keeping your arms straight, elbows slightly bent, slowly raise the weights out to your sides until your arms are parallel to the floor. Pause for 1 second at the top of the move, slowly lower your arms to your sides, and repeat.

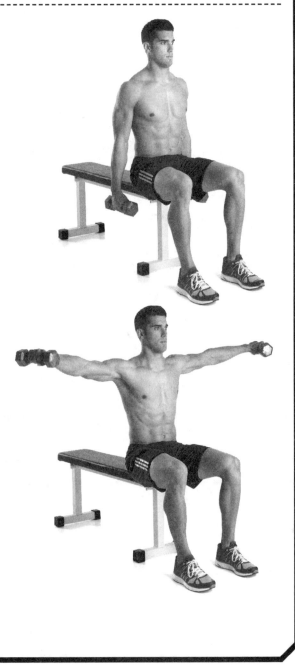

★ TRAINER'S TIP

Don't grab the same weights you typically use when performing this exercise from a standing position. Staying seated makes it more difficult to swing the weight up using momentum, which is what most guys do when trying the exercise standing. Try picking a weight that's roughly 40 to 50 percent lighter to start.

SEATED LATERAL RAISE/ LATERAL RAISE AND HOLD SUPERSET

MUSCLES TARGETED:
medial deltoids

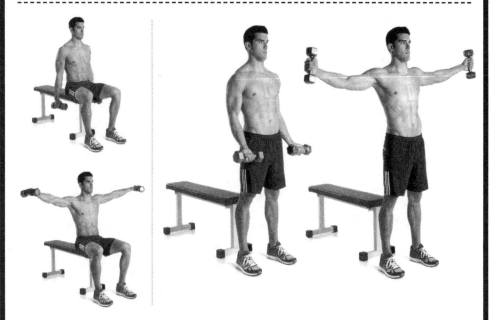

This superset is a combination of two exercises described elsewhere in this book:
the seated lateral raise and the lateral raise and hold.

START POSITION

➜ Sit on an exercise bench with a light dumbbell in each hand and your feet flat on the floor. Your arms should hang straight down at your sides with your palms facing in toward each other.

THE MOVE: Keeping your arms straight, elbows slightly bent, slowly raise the weights out to your sides until your arms are parallel to the floor. Pause for 1 second at the top of the move, slowly lower your arms to your sides, and repeat for the required number of repetitions.

    Immediately afterward, pop off the bench and stand straight, holding a dumbbell in each hand, with your arms hanging down at your sides, palms facing forward. Without twisting your wrists, raise the weights up until your arms are parallel to the floor, then hold that position for the required amount of time.

★ TRAINER'S TIP

Don't use the same pair of dumbbells for both exercises if you feel one of the moves isn't challenging enough. Instead, pick the right pair for each exercise to hit your muscles evenly.

SEATED MILITARY PRESS
(OVERLOAD)

MUSCLES TARGETED:
shoulders and triceps

START POSITION

➜ Sit on a weight bench facing the barbell rack with your feet flat on the floor. Grab the bar in front of you with hands slightly more than shoulder-width apart and rest it just across the top of your chest.

THE MOVE: Press the bar up above your head until your arms are straight, elbows locked. Pause, then slowly lower the bar straight down until it lightly touches the top of your head. Explosively press the weight back above you until your arms are straight, and repeat.

★ TRAINER'S TIP

The object of this exercise is twofold. It's designed to improve your strength within a limited range of motion, as well as work your muscles through a straight up-and-down motion they normally never achieve when you use a barbell. That's because most men lower the bar to their chest or to the back of their neck, which slightly changes the angle of the arms.

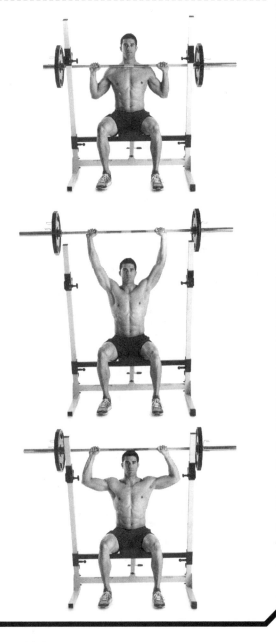

SHOULDER BOX

MUSCLES TARGETED:
shoulders

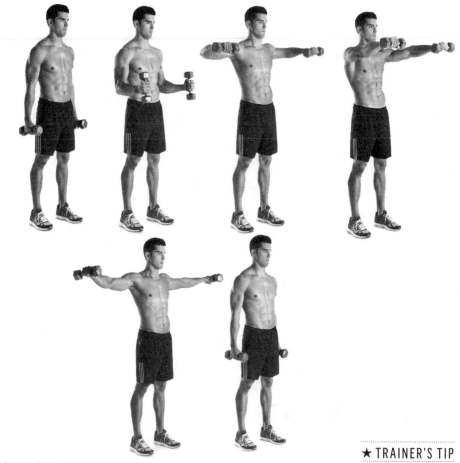

START POSITION

➡ Stand straight with a light dumbbell in each hand and your arms hanging down at your sides, palms facing in.

THE MOVE: Curl the weights halfway up until your forearms are parallel to the floor—your arms should form 90-degree angles. Keeping your arms at 90 degrees, raise your elbows up and out from your sides until your upper arms are parallel to the floor. Push the weights out in front of you until your arms are straight and parallel to the floor, palms facing down. Keeping your arms straight, sweep them straight back until they are in line with your upper back—you should look like the letter T from the front. Lower your arms to your sides. Repeat the five-step move for the duration of the exercise.

★ TRAINER'S TIP
Don't be concerned with how much weight you're using with this prehab exercise—it's a proactive move designed to prevent postural and muscular imbalances that could lead to shoulder injuries when performing more complex moves for building your chest, shoulders, and triceps.

SIDE ISO AB

MUSCLES TARGETED:
obliques, core

START POSITION

➜ Lie on your left side with your upper body propped up on your left forearm—your upper arm should be perpendicular to the floor so that your left elbow is directly below your left shoulder, fist pointing forward.

THE MOVE: Keeping your upper body steady, slowly push your hips up until your body is in a straight line from your feet to your shoulders. Hold for the prescribed amount of time, then switch positions to work the opposite side.

★ TRAINER'S TIP

If this move is too difficult to hold for the required amount of time, hold the pose for as long as possible and rest for 2 or 3 seconds; continue this pattern until you reach the target time.

SINGLE-ARM CABLE PUSHDOWN

MUSCLES TARGETED:
triceps

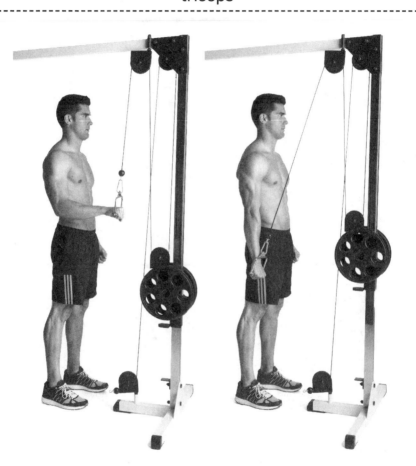

START POSITION

➜ Attach a handle to a high-cable pulley and grab it with an overhand grip with your right hand. Tuck your upper arm into your side and stand with your back straight, feet shoulder-width apart.

THE MOVE: Without moving your upper arm, press the handle straight down until your right arm is extended, elbow locked, with your fist down by your thigh. Raise the handle back to the start position and repeat for the required number of repetitions. Afterward, switch positions to work your left arm.

★ TRAINER'S TIP

Your wrist should stay in line with your forearm—don't let your knuckles pull back toward your elbow. Doing so displaces some of the stress of the move onto your wrists instead of your triceps.

STANDING OVERHEAD PRESS

MUSCLES TARGETED:
shoulders and triceps

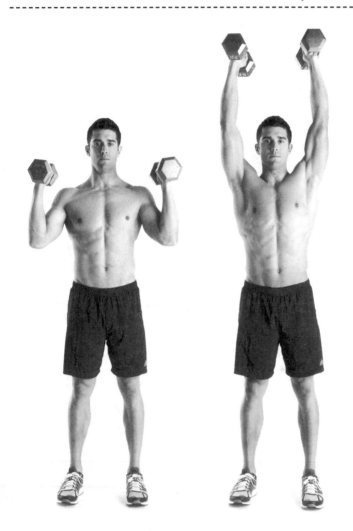

START POSITION

➜ With your feet shoulder-width apart, stand straight holding a dumbbell in each hand above shoulder level with a neutral grip (palms facing each other).

THE MOVE: Keeping your back straight and eyes looking forward, press the weights up over your head until your arms are straight, elbows locked. Lower the weights to your shoulders, and repeat.

★ TRAINER'S TIP

The weights should travel in a straight line starting from your shoulders. Don't press them toward each other as if the goal were to allow the dumbbells to touch at the top of the movement.

TRICEPS KICKBACK

MUSCLES TARGETED:
triceps

START POSITION

➜ Stand with your left side to the exercise bench and a light dumbbell in your right hand. Rest your left hand and knee on the bench, letting your right arm hang below you, palm facing in. Pull your elbow up until your upper arm is parallel to the floor.

THE MOVE: Keeping your upper arm stationary, extend your right arm back behind you until it's straight, elbow locked. Pause for 2 seconds, then bend your elbow to lower the weight back into the start position, and repeat. Afterward, switch positions to work your left arm.

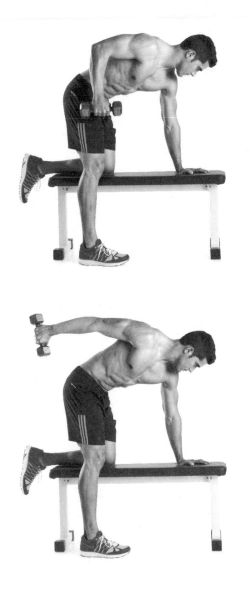

★ TRAINER'S TIP

Keep your head in line with your back by staring straight down at the bench. Don't make the mistake of turning your head to check in a mirror whether your arm is straight, since this can sometimes cause neck stress. Instead, look to make sure your upper arm is parallel to the floor before you start the exercise, then continue to stare down at the bench for the remainder of the movement.

45-DEGREE BENT-OVER ROW

MUSCLES TARGETED:

latissimus dorsi, middle trapezius, and lower back

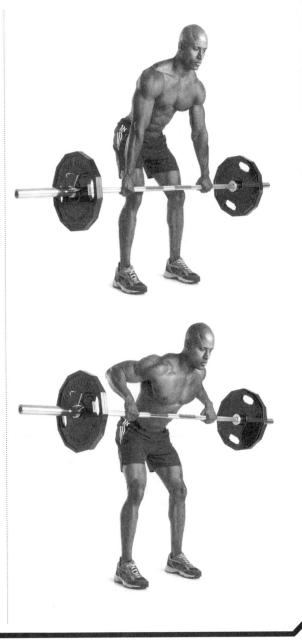

START POSITION

→ Stand behind a barbell with your feet shoulder-width apart. Bend at the waist and grab the bar with an overhand grip, hands slightly more than shoulder-width apart. Lift the barbell off the floor and stand straight. Bending at your hips, lower your torso about halfway from parallel to the floor—your torso should be at a 45-degree angle. Allow your arms to hang straight down.

THE MOVE: Keeping your back and legs locked in this position, quickly pull the bar up until it touches your midsection. Lower the weight until your arms are straight, and repeat.

★ TRAINER'S TIP

A common mistake men make when performing this exercise is failing to keep their torso at a 45-degree angle.

Instead of focusing on the bar, pay close attention to keeping your back fixed throughout the exercise. Any time you feel your torso rise, you're using momentum to jerk the weight upward, which is cheating and may cause injury.

BENT-OVER BARBELL ROW

MUSCLES TARGETED:

latissimus dorsi, middle trapezius, and lower back

START POSITION

➜ Stand behind a barbell with your feet shoulder-width apart. Bend at the waist and grab the bar with an overhand grip, hands slightly wider than shoulder-width. Lift the barbell off the floor and position your torso so it's slightly above parallel to the floor. (Your arms should hang straight below you.)

THE MOVE: Keeping your back flat and legs slightly bent, quickly pull the bar up until it touches your midsection right between your lower chest and your belly button. Slowly lower it until your arms are straight, and repeat.

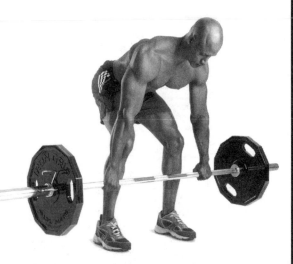

★ TRAINER'S TIP

Don't lock your knees—keep them slightly bent throughout the move.

DEADLIFT

trapezius, lower back, hamstrings, and glutes

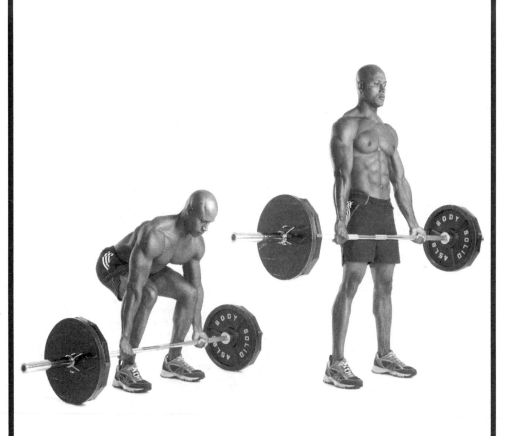

START POSITION

➜ Stand facing a barbell with the bar over your toes, feet hip-width apart. Bend your knees and grasp the bar with an alternating grip (one hand pronated, one hand supinated) and your hands shoulder-width apart.

THE MOVE: With your chest up and back flat, stand up (keeping the bar close to your body as you lift) until your legs are straight, knees unlocked. Pause, lower the bar to the floor, then repeat.

★ TRAINER'S TIP

Make sure to keep your arms straight during the exercise and resist the urge to raise your shoulders or bend your elbows as you go.

DECLINE BENCH REVERSE CRUNCH

MUSCLES TARGETED:
rectus abdominis

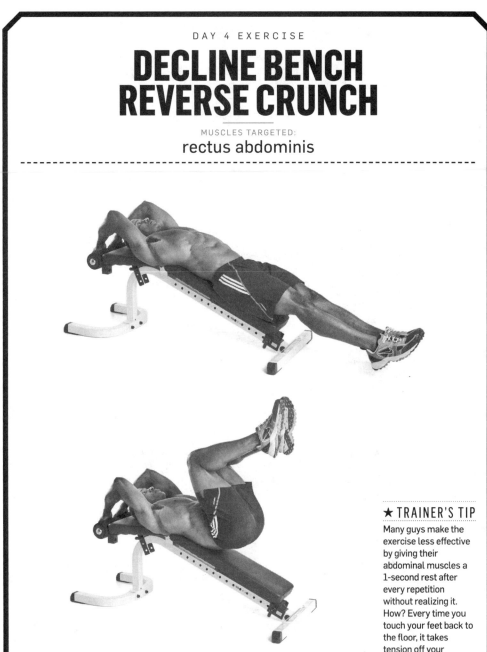

START POSITION

➜ Lie down on a decline situp board with your head resting at the higher end. Reach back, grab the top of the bench, and flatten your head and back against the bench. Extend your legs straight in front of you.

THE MOVE: Tighten your core muscles, then draw your knees up to your chest. Pause, then extend your legs back into the start position, and repeat.

★ TRAINER'S TIP

Many guys make the exercise less effective by giving their abdominal muscles a 1-second rest after every repetition without realizing it. How? Every time you touch your feet back to the floor, it takes tension off your muscles and gives them a breather. Instead, leave your heels raised just above the floor the entire time—it keeps your abs contracted and maximizes your results.

DUMBBELL PULLOVER

MUSCLES TARGETED:
latissimus dorsi and middle trapezius

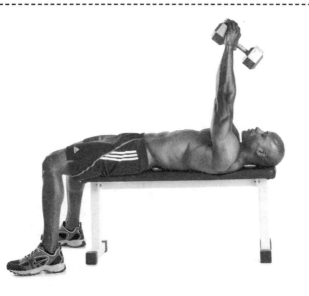

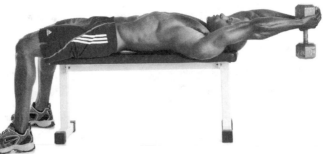

START POSITION

➜ Grab a dumbbell and lie back on a flat bench with your feet flat on the floor. Shift yourself so that the top of your head is at the very end. Hold the dumbbell end over end on your chest, wrapping your thumbs and forefingers in a diamond shape right below the top bell. Press the weight over your chest, leaving your elbows slightly bent.

THE MOVE: Keeping your arms fixed in a slightly bent position, slowly lower the weight backward in an arc over your head until your upper arms are in line with your head. Pause, pull the weight back into the start position over your chest, then repeat.

★ TRAINER'S TIP

Your arms should never bend or straighten as you perform the exercise—if they do, you're cheating by adding your triceps muscles into the mix.

DUMBBELL SHRUG

MUSCLES TARGETED:
upper trapezius

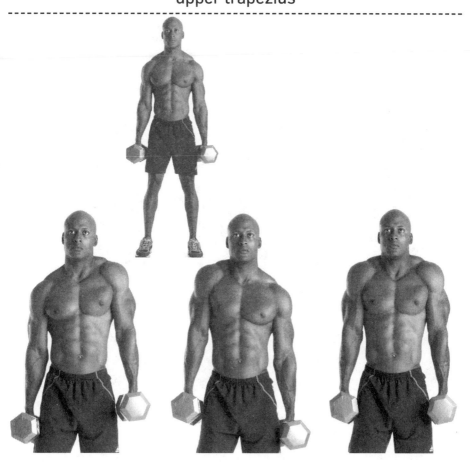

★ TRAINER'S TIP

Keep your arms straight at all times. Also, avoid rotating and/or rolling your shoulders as you lift the weight. Your upper trapezius muscles are designed to pull your shoulders up and down—not backward or forward—so doing this increases your odds of straining your neck muscles.

START POSITION

➜ Stand straight, holding a heavy dumbbell in each hand, arms hanging down at your sides, palms facing in.

THE MOVE: Without moving your right arm, raise your left shoulder up to your ear as high as you can. Lower it, then repeat, this time raising your right shoulder only. Lower and repeat a final time, this time raising both shoulders at the same time. Continue the pattern (left, right, and both) for the duration of the set.

FARMER'S WALK

MUSCLES TARGETED:

legs, calves, traps, and forearms

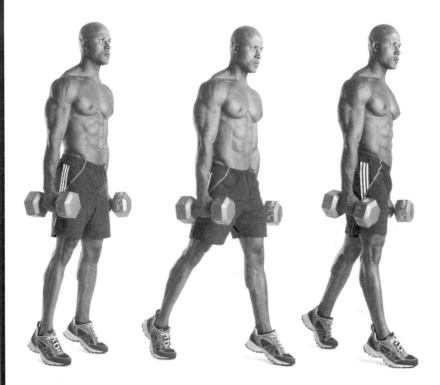

★ TRAINER'S TIP

Focus on your feet. Paying attention to the weights may cause you to lift them by raising your shoulders, which will exhaust your upper body before you thoroughly train your calves. Also, if you lack enough space to walk around in, you can walk in either a circle or a figure-eight.

START POSITION

→ Stand straight, holding a heavy dumbbell in each hand, letting your arms hang down straight at your sides. Raise your heels off the floor so you're balancing on the balls of your feet.

THE MOVE: Keeping your heels off the floor, walk forward on the balls of your feet for the required distance.

HANGING SPREAD-V LEG RAISE

MUSCLES TARGETED:
abdominals and core

START POSITION

➜ Hang from a chinup bar with your hands spaced more than shoulder-width apart. Your legs should be slightly bent underneath you, your legs and feet together.

THE MOVE: Keeping your legs and feet together, raise your legs up until they are parallel to the floor. Pause, then spread your legs apart as wide as you can. Pause, then bring your legs back together, keeping them parallel to the floor. Pause a final time, then lower your legs into the start position.

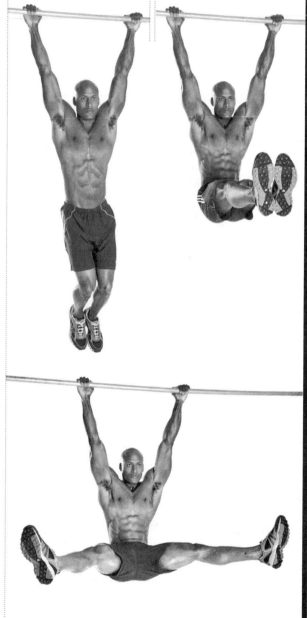

★ TRAINER'S TIP

Make sure you pause for a second with each transition within the exercise. This tweak makes the exercise more challenging by keeping continuous tension on your abs, as well as by eliminating as much assistance as possible from any momentum that can occur as you raise and lower your legs.

MEDICINE-BALL SMASH

MUSCLES TARGETED:
upper back and core

This is an alternate exercise
to the Sledgehammer.

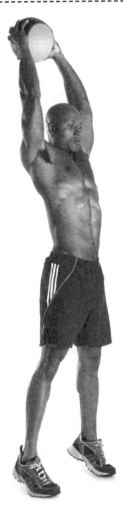
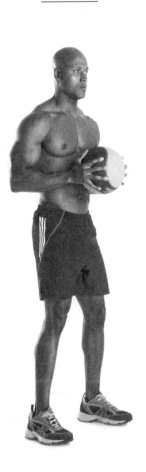

START POSITION

➜ Grab a heavy medicine ball that doesn't bounce. Stand straight with your feet shoulder-width apart, holding the ball with both hands in front of you.

THE MOVE: Quickly raise the ball directly over your head and rise up on your toes as far as possible. Keeping your arms straight, quickly lower them as you bend at the waist and slam the ball down onto the floor directly in front of you. Pick up the ball, and repeat.

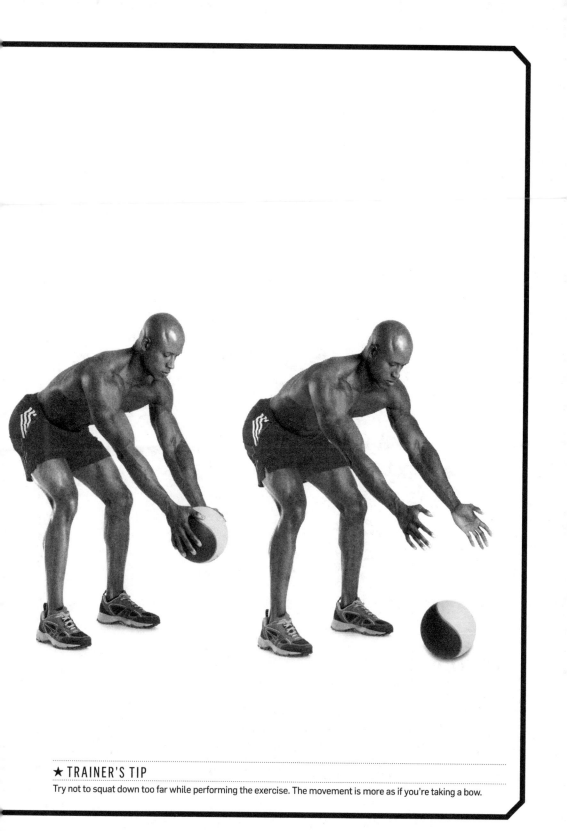

★ TRAINER'S TIP

Try not to squat down too far while performing the exercise. The movement is more as if you're taking a bow.

TESTOSTERONE **229** TRANSFORMATION

OVERHEAD BARBELL SIDE BENDS

MUSCLES TARGETED:

core

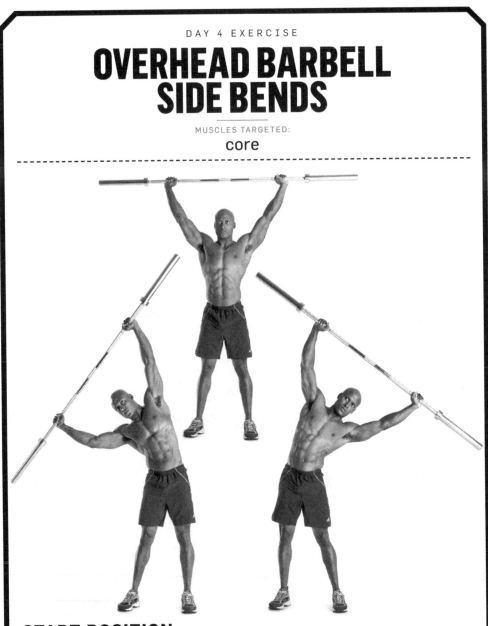

START POSITION

➜ Grab a bar (one with no weight plates on it) with a firm overhand grip, hands more than shoulder-width apart. Press the bar directly over your head until your arms are straight, elbows unlocked.

THE MOVE: Maintaining a tight grip on the bar, bend at your waist and lean to your right as far as you comfortably can. Don't twist at the waist or bend your arms as you go. Return to the start position, then immediately lean to the left. Continue to alternate from right to left for the required number of repetitions.

★ TRAINER'S TIP

Don't expect a big range of motion in this exercise. The movement will seem extremely slight, but it's a very effective tool for making sure your body is strong through every plane of motion.

REVERSE SHRUG

MUSCLES TARGETED:
upper back and trapezius

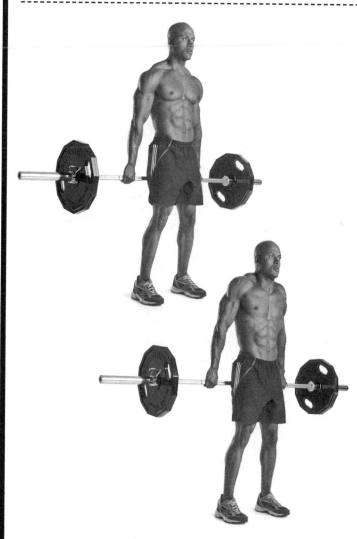

START POSITION

➡ Stand straight, holding a barbell directly behind you with an overhand grip, hands shoulder-width apart—your palms should end up facing behind you. Let your arms hang straight down at your sides.

THE MOVE: Without bending your arms, raise your shoulders straight up as high as you can. Pause, lower, and repeat.

★ TRAINER'S TIP

Getting the bar in position behind your body can be the hardest part of the exercise. That's where having access to a power rack or a spotter is essential. But if you don't have either, simply reverse the bar racks on a standard bench (so that the lower portion faces away from the bench), then lower them down as far as possible. Place the bar on the racks, stand with your back facing the bar, and grab it from there.

SIDE MEDICINE-BALL TOSS

MUSCLES TARGETED:
upper back and core

START POSITION

➜ Step about 3 feet away from a wall sturdy enough to hit with a medicine ball (brick or concrete will do) and stand perpendicular to it so that your right shoulder faces the wall. Your knees should be slightly bent, your feet shoulder-width apart. Grab a medicine ball with both hands and extend your arms out so they're straight and parallel to the floor.

THE MOVE: Keeping your arms straight, rotate to the left, then quickly rotate to the right, pivoting your feet so that your toes turn to face the wall as you go—and release the ball as hard as possible at the wall. Catch the rebound, rotate your body back into the start position, and repeat. After performing the required number of repetitions, repeat the exercise, this time standing perpendicular to the wall so that your left shoulder faces it.

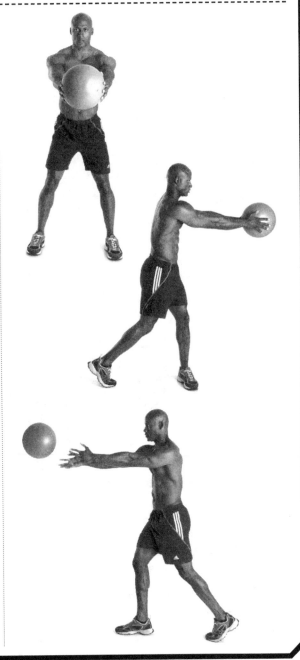

★ TRAINER'S TIP

Never bend your arms as you throw the ball to try and toss it harder—all of the power should come from the rotation of your body instead.

SINGLE-ARM DUMBBELL ROW

MUSCLES TARGETED:

latissimus dorsi, lower back, and rhomboids

START POSITION

➜ Stand with your left side to a flat bench, with a dumbbell in your left hand. Rest your left hand and knee on the bench, bend at the waist, and let your right arm hang down toward the floor, palm facing in toward the bench.

THE MOVE: Powerfully draw the weight up close to your body until it reaches the outside of your chest. Lower the weight until your arm is straight, and repeat. After you've finished the required number of repetitions, switch positions to work your left arm.

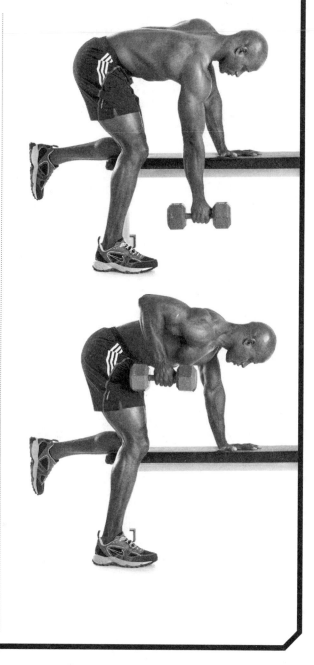

★ TRAINER'S TIP

As you row, imagine that the goal is to raise your elbow up to the ceiling, instead of pulling the weight with your hand. Also, don't twist your torso as you row. Your lower-back and core muscles will take on some of the effort, preventing you from pre-exhausting your upper lats.

SINGLE-ARM LOW-CABLE ROW

MUSCLES TARGETED:

latissimus dorsi, lower back, and rhomboids

START POSITION

➡ Attach a single handle to a low-cable pulley station. Stand about 3 feet from the cable machine and grab the handle with your right hand. Bend your knees and lean back so that your torso is at an angle, with your right arm extended straight out in front of you, palm facing to the side—your left hand can rest on your left thigh for balance.

THE MOVE: Holding this posture, pull the handle straight back until it reaches your right side. Return the handle to the start position and repeat for the required number of repetitions. After you've finished, switch positions to work your left side.

★ TRAINER'S TIP

You'll know if you're leaning back far enough at the start of the move if you feel you could pull the weight back toward you without pulling yourself off-balance or forward.

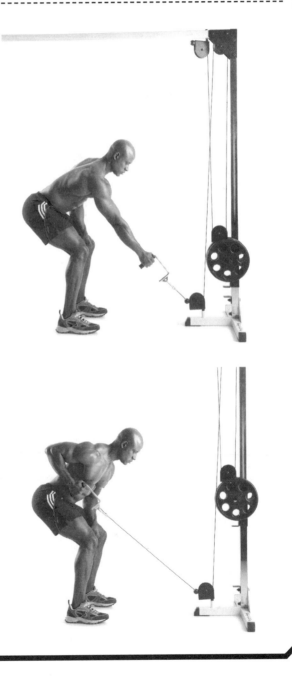

SLED DRAG

MUSCLES TARGETED:

hamstrings, lower back, glutes, and calves

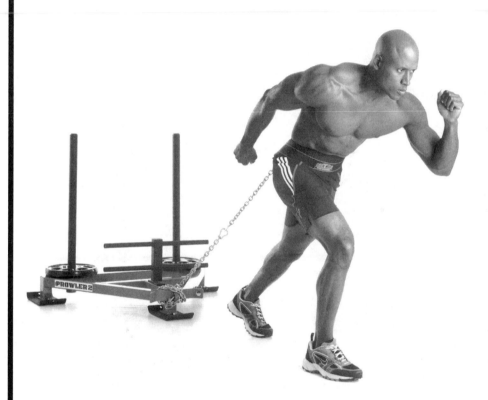

★ TRAINER'S TIP

If you run out of room as you go, simply turn around by making a wide circle and travel back the opposite way. Also, focus on your hips, not your feet: The less they wiggle as you go—as if you're using a Hula-Hoop—the better your form will be (and the greater the results).

START POSITION

➜ Stand with the weight belt strapped around your waist, arms down at your sides. Lean forward into a slightly bent-over position (body in front of feet).

THE MOVE: Begin to quickly run forward. Keep your chest up and your back arched as you go—don't round your back. (You should feel the move on your hips, not your spine.) Pull for the required 60 seconds, rest for 1 to 2 minutes, then repeat.

SLEDGEHAMMER

MUSCLES TARGETED:

core, upper back, glutes, hip adductors and abductors, forearms, and hands (grip)

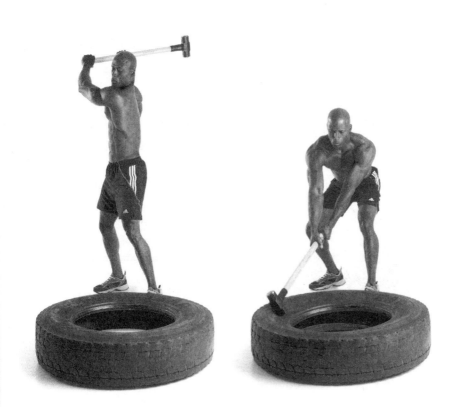

If performing this exercise is impossible for you due to space or availability of equipment, perform the medicine-ball smash (page 228) instead.

START POSITION

➜ Place a large truck tire on the floor and stand approximately 18 inches away from it in a staggered stance—left foot in front of your right—keeping a slight bend in your knees. Grab the sledgehammer tight with both hands. Then, twist your upper body (not your hips) to the right to position the hammer behind you, over your right shoulder.

THE MOVE: Rotate your torso to the left as you swing the hammer down toward the inside lip of the tire. As you swing, your top hand should slide down the handle toward your bottom hand so that when you hit the tire, your hands are stacked one above the other. Reverse the motion by

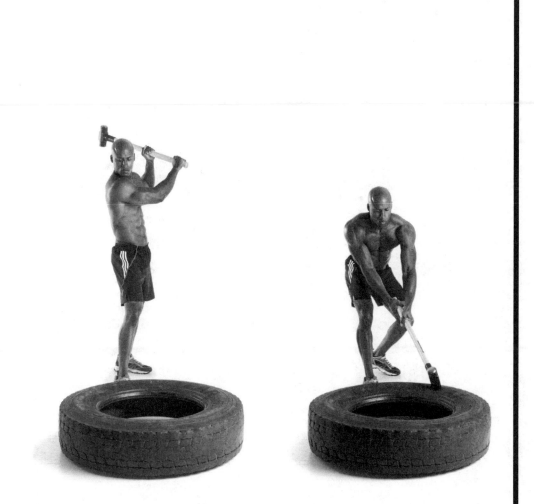

rotating your upper body to the right—letting your right hand slide back to the start position—and repeat. After you've finished the required amount of time, switch positions to work the opposite side.

Finally, stand about 2 feet from the tire with your feet shoulder-width apart and parallel to each other. Grab the very end of the sledgehammer with both hands together. Raise the hammer straight up over your head, then swing it down in front of you and hit the tire. Repeat for the required amount of time.

★ TRAINER'S TIP
This classic exercise is ideal for training your trunk to transfer power, an advantage that will allow you to lift more weight.

SNATCH HIGH PULL

MUSCLES TARGETED:
full body

This is an alternate to the Tire Flip exercise for those who don't have access to a large truck tire.

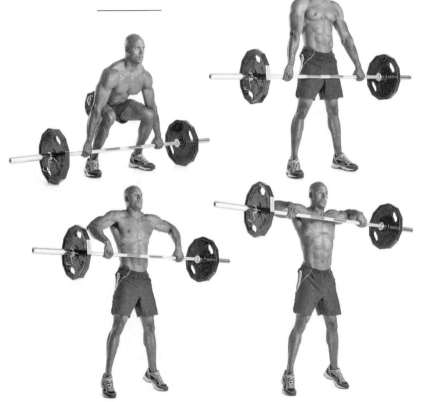

START POSITION

➡ Stand in front of a barbell with your feet shoulder-width apart. Squat down and grab the bar with an overhand grip, your hands spaced as wide as you can comfortably grab.

THE MOVE: This exercise has two pulls—one to get the bar off the floor and another to move the bar up to your chest. For the first pull, quickly stand up to raise the bar to the middle of your thighs. For the second pull, immediately press through the balls of your feet—raising your heels as you go—and quickly yank the bar up to your chest by shrugging your shoulders and bending your arms. (Imagine you're trying to toss the bar toward the ceiling.) Lower the barbell to the start position and repeat for the required number of repetitions.

★ TRAINER'S TIP

Although the exercise is described as two parts, it is actually meant to be performed in one continuous motion. There is no pause between pulls. As soon as you lift the bar off the floor, you'll immediately shrug your shoulders and pull it up toward your chest.

STRAIGHT-ARM PULLDOWN

MUSCLES TARGETED:
latissimus dorsi

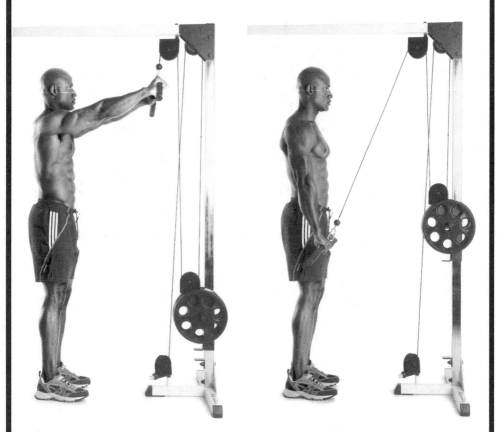

START POSITION

➜ Stand a few feet in front of a high-cable pulley, feet slightly more than hip-width apart for stability. Reach up and grab the bar with an overhand grip, hands slightly more than shoulder-width apart.

THE MOVE: With your arms straight, slowly lower the bar down in front of you until it touches the front of your thighs. Slowly raise the bar back into the start position, and repeat.

★ **TRAINER'S TIP**
Don't bend your arms or lean forward as you go. You want your back muscles—not your chest or triceps—to pull the bar downward.

T-BAR ROW

MUSCLES TARGETED:

back, middle and lower trapezius, rhomboids

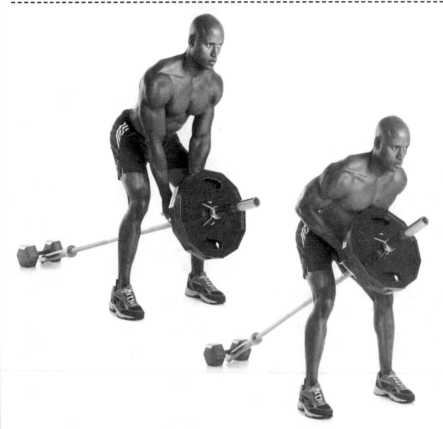

START POSITION

➜ Place one end of an Olympic barbell in the corner of the room at an angle or under the handle of a heavy dumbbell. Load the other end up with a few weight plates, then straddle the bar so that you're facing the weight plates. Place a V-grip handle (the kind that positions your palms so that they face each other) underneath the bar and grab a handle in each hand. Bend your knees, then bend forward at your waist so that your torso is at a 45-degree angle. Your arms should be extended below you, your head in line with your back.

THE MOVE: Keeping your back flat, pull the bar up toward your chest. Pause, lower the bar back to the start position, then repeat.

★ TRAINER'S TIP

As in the land mine, if you don't have a corner in which to place the bar—or don't want to scuff up your walls—you can create a corner by positioning two heavy dumbbells next to each other or even use one as shown. This will keep the bar in place.

TIRE FLIP

MUSCLES TARGETED:
full body

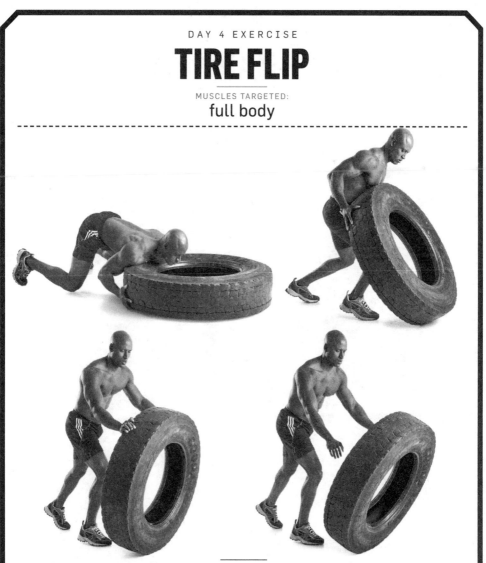

To do this exercise, you'll need a large truck tire and some space to flip it.
If you don't have a tire, perform the snatch high pull on page 238 instead.

START POSITION

➡ Squat down about 18 to 24 inches from the tire. Lean forward and
place your hands underneath the bottom of the tire with your hands
more than shoulder-width apart. Make sure your heels are up in the air
so that your weight rests on the balls of your feet.

THE MOVE: Driving forward through your legs, push the tire up and
forward as fast as possible. If you like, you can use your knee to help flip
the tire over or push hard with both hands. Once the tire lands, resume
the start position and repeat.

★ TRAINER'S TIP
If you're in the right
position at the start of
the move, your chin
should be close to
touching the top edge
of the tire, your chest
buried into the side of
the tire.

TRAP-BAR SHRUG

MUSCLES TARGETED:
trapezius

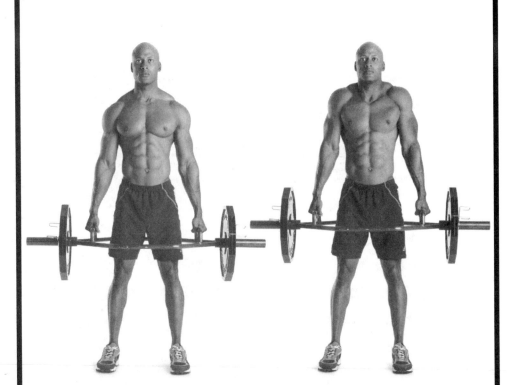

To perform this power exercise, you'll need a trap bar—a specialized bar that you can hold using a neutral grip—with your palms facing each other.

START POSITION

➜ Step into the center of a trap bar with plates loaded, squat down, and grab the handles. Rise up so that you're standing straight with your feet hip-width apart.

THE MOVE: Keeping your arms straight—resist the urge to bend them at the elbow—raise your shoulders up as high as you can. Pause, lower, and repeat.

★ TRAINER'S TIP
The reason this move is so vital for T-boosting is that it allows you to use more weight than you would normally handle performing the exercise with either a barbell or a pair of dumbbells.

WEIGHTED CHINUP

MUSCLES TARGETED:

latissimus dorsi, rhomboids, lower trapezius, biceps, and forearms

For this exercise, you'll need a weighted vest or a dip belt. If you don't have one, you can also have a training partner place a dumbbell between your legs just above the knees, or wedged between your ankles, as shown. Then brace it there by squeezing your legs together.

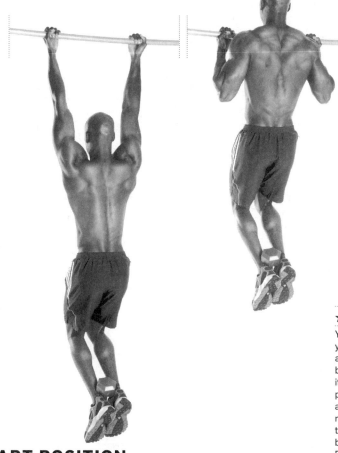

★ TRAINER'S TIP

Your biceps can help your back lift greater amounts of weight for bigger gains. However, if you don't pull properly with your arms, they will do more of the work and tire out before your back muscles do. Before you begin the exercise, draw your shoulder blades back first to contract your back muscles—this will help align your body so your back does the bulk of the work.

START POSITION

➜ Grab the bar with a supinated grip (palms facing you) with your hands slightly more than shoulder-width apart. Hang from the bar with your arms straight, elbows unlocked.

THE MOVE: Quickly pull yourself up until the bar is directly under your chest, then lower yourself back down, and repeat.

WEIGHTED CHINUP 21

MUSCLES TARGETED:

latissimus dorsi, rhomboids, lower trapezius, biceps, and forearms

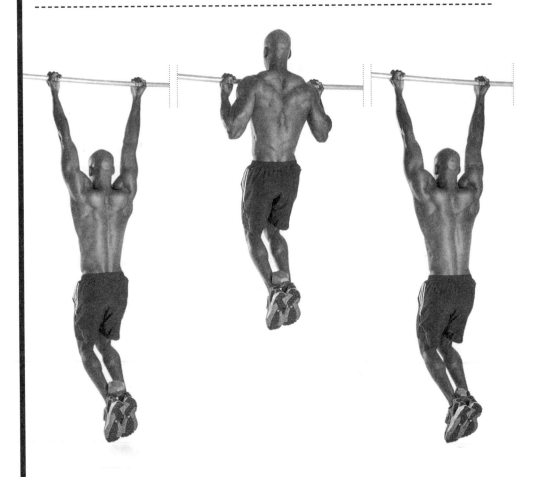

START POSITION

➡ Grab the bar with a supinated grip (palms facing you), with your hands slightly more than shoulder-width apart. Have a partner place the dumbbell between your legs just above the knees—or wedged between your ankles as shown—and hold it there. Hang from the bar with your arms straight, elbows unlocked.

THE MOVE: Slowly pull yourself up until the bar is directly under your chest, slowly lower yourself back down, and repeat for 7 reps. Without letting go of the bar, have your partner replace the dumbbell with a lighter one, then do 7 more reps. Finally, drop the light dumbbell (so you're lifting only your body weight) and finish the exercise by completing 7 more reps.

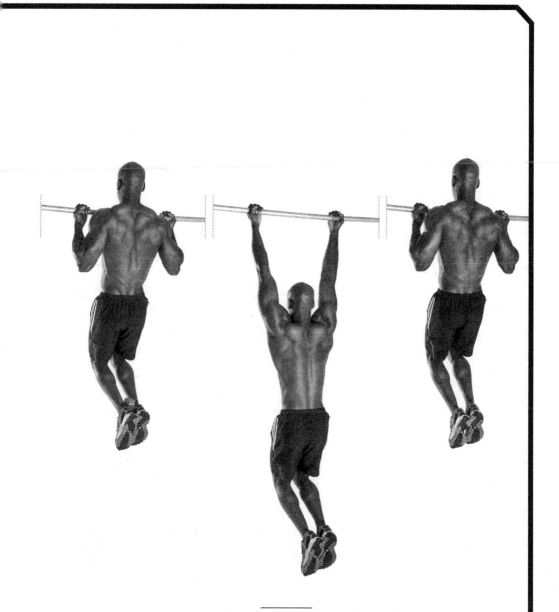

For this exercise, you'll need two dumbbells—one that will help you exhaust your muscles within 10 reps, and then a lighter one about half that weight.

★ TRAINER'S TIP

If you don't have a partner, you can add weight yourself by purchasing a pair of 15-pound chains, but if you're not that strong, you can use lighter ones. That way, instead of having to hold a dumbbell with your feet, simply drape both chains around your neck at the start of the move.

YATES ROW

MUSCLES TARGETED:
back and biceps

START POSITION

➡ Grab a barbell with an underhand grip and stand with your feet shoulder-width apart and your knees slightly bent. Bend at your hips, lowering your torso about 20 to 25 degrees, and letting the bar hang straight down from your shoulders.

THE MOVE: Keeping your back and legs locked in this position, slowly pull the bar up until it touches your midsection. Lower the weight until your arms are straight, and repeat.

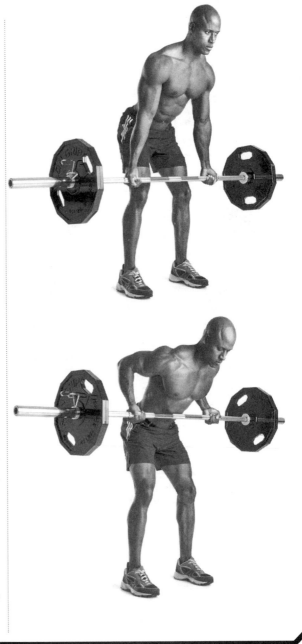

★ TRAINER'S TIP

Unlike a normal bent-over row—or even the 45-degree bent-over row that you'll also perform in this 12-week routine—the Yates row uses a smaller range of motion to target the back, so don't expect to move the bar that far up or down. Don't lean back once you've pulled the weight up. Instead, stay as strict with your form as possible and you'll feel—and see—the difference this mass-building, T-elevating move can make.

YOUR MUSCLE GUIDE

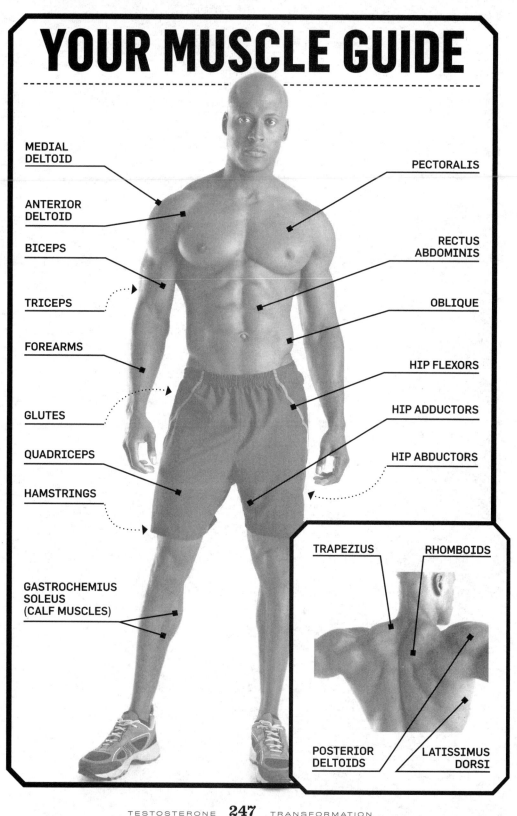

MEDIAL
DELTOID

ANTERIOR
DELTOID

BICEPS

TRICEPS

FOREARMS

GLUTES

QUADRICEPS

HAMSTRINGS

GASTROCHEMIUS
SOLEUS
(CALF MUSCLES)

PECTORALIS

RECTUS
ABDOMINIS

OBLIQUE

HIP FLEXORS

HIP ADDUCTORS

HIP ABDUCTORS

TRAPEZIUS

RHOMBOIDS

POSTERIOR
DELTOIDS

LATISSIMUS
DORSI

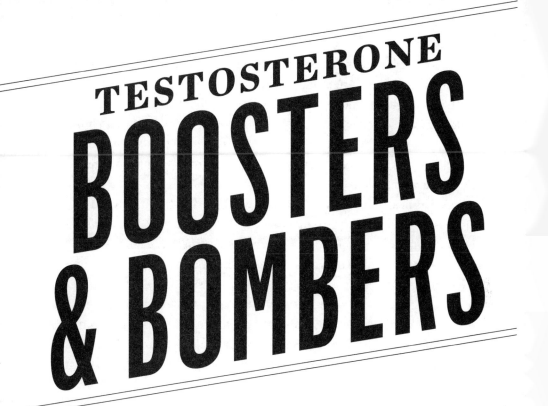

TESTOSTERONE
BOOSTERS
& BOMBERS

Lifestyle changes that can elevate testosterone and improve your fitness and health

CHAPTER

14

I used to know a guy at the gym who was an animal in the weight room. He attacked the barbell with the intensity of a 5-year-old ripping into a birthday present.

Unlike a lot of guys, he didn't waste time talking to friends or messing with the music on the gym's stereo. Once his workout started, he was focused—moving from barbell to notebook to barbell to notebook, a three-ring binder that held his workout charts and progress logs. He'd spend at least an hour and a half lifting, sometimes 2 hours, 4 to 5 days a week. And he'd end every session the same way: crack a raw egg into a shaker of protein drink and down it with a turkey sandwich.

This guy was pretty strong, and his body was lean, but he didn't have the muscle mass you'd expect from someone who hit the weights as hard as he did. I couldn't figure it out. He lifted heavy. His routine was even more intense than mine. Why was I getting bigger when he was staying the same?

Then one night when I was out late with some friends, I saw him tending bar at a club. Later, some guys at the gym told me that he moonlighted there a couple of nights a week and that he liked to party hard on his nights off. It all made sense. The squat-rack workhorse played hard (and didn't get much sleep). He was burning his candle at both ends, and probably in the middle, too—and undermining his efforts in the gym in the process. If you want to lower your testosterone, nothing works better than the one-two punch of inadequate shut-eye and shots of tequila. But other lifestyle choices influence T-levels and muscle building, too. Many of the simplest decisions that you make every day can secretly have a hand in either boosting your testosterone or slowing it down—or, even worse, stopping it in its tracks. To help yourself reap the benefits of optimum testosterone, examine your life for ways to embrace the following T-Boosters and minimize the T-Bombers.

THE TESTOSTERONE BOOSTERS

T-BOOSTER: GOOD SLEEP

As I mentioned at the beginning of this book, the pursuit of the Great American Lifestyle has left many men more sleep-deprived than ever. (And that was part of my gym buddy's problem.) Getting less-than-adequate sleep steals critical recovery time away from your workout-stressed muscles and sabotages the 8-hour window during which your body releases its greatest amounts of both testosterone and growth hormone.

A 2011 study performed at the University of Chicago found that getting only 5 hours of sleep—instead of the recommended 8 hours a night—decreased men's testosterone levels by 10 to 15 percent. After allowing 10 young men to sleep for 3 days for up to 10 hours under laboratory conditions, researchers forced them to sleep just 5 hours a night for 8 straight nights. The result: Not only did their T-levels plummet, but so did their mood and energy. Ever try to get a good workout when you're feeling lethargic and bummed out? It's not going to happen.

All-Day Testosterone: Although sleep experts recommend at least 7 to 8 hours each night to manage levels of cortisol—a stress hormone that can rise when you're sleep-deprived and disrupt testosterone production—aim for more (up to 10 hours, if possible). That goes double if you still find yourself constantly tired or don't feel as if your body is fully recovered the day after a workout. If getting more than 8 hours is impossible, then try to sneak a 20-to-30-minute nap somewhere in the middle of your day. You'll get a surge of hormones, plus it can help you relax enough to lower your cortisol levels.

T-BOOSTER: BELLY BREATHING

Most men, certainly those with Type-A personalities, tend to chest-breathe; that is, they take short, quick breaths that don't utilize the full capacity of their lungs. Upper-chest breathing goes hand in hand with stress, agitation, and anxiety. And it increases your body's output of T-crashing cortisol. But you can learn to counteract that—and relax—with simple breathing lessons. A study performed by Spain's renowned University of the Basque Country found that when subjects performed a type of voluntary breathing therapy called diaphragmatic breathing, their cortisol levels noticeably decreased.

All-Day Testosterone: At least twice a day—or as often as possible—sit in a quiet place, free of distractions, close your eyes, and breathe slowly and deeply for 5 to 10 minutes. To do it right, place one hand on your chest and the other on your belly. As you breathe deeply, allow your belly to inflate before your chest rises. This brings oxygen deep into the lower half of your lungs. Don't let your chest rise—instead breathe through your diaphragm, letting your belly inflate and deflate. This tactic—known as diaphragmatic breathing—reduces stress, relaxes the body and mind, and has been shown to reduce the amount of free radicals (the molecules responsible for aging and tissue damage) that are left in your system after exercise. A study by the Department of Experimental Medicine and Public Health at the University of Camerino, in Italy, took athletes who had finished an exhaustive training session and broke them into two groups. The first concentrated on their breathing in a quiet place, while the second group simply sat in a quiet place. Not only were cortisol levels lower in the group that spent time performing diaphragmatic breathing, but they also experienced a reduction in exercise-induced oxidative stress (fewer free radicals) and a boost in melatonin, a hormone that assists in everything from keeping your sleep cycles on schedule to preventing muscle damage during long, intense workouts.

T-BOOSTER: BACKING A WINNER

Rooting for the underdog is something a lot of guys love to do. But always cheering for the loser may be the reason you're losing in the T-level department—especially if they almost never win.

When researchers at Duke University and the University of Michigan monitored the T-levels of a group of men and women before and after the 2008 election, they found that the testosterone levels in women didn't change after the returns came in, even if their candidate had lost.

But when it came to the men, they experienced an immediate change in their testosterone after the election results were announced. The T-levels in men who voted for Obama remained stable and didn't fall as much as T-levels typically do during certain times of the day. However, men who voted for McCain experienced an immediate drop in their T-levels.

All-Day Testosterone: Pick a winner. Are you an alumnus of a high school or college that has a top-ranked football or basketball team? Does your favorite NFL, NBA, NHL, or MLB team have a shot to win it all this year? Following a winning team during the season may keep T-levels high. Studies have shown that winning increases testosterone, while losing reduces it. It may be that the effect is due to changes in dominance and personal status or ranking. Experiments that tested testosterone levels in saliva have found that T rises or falls in response to changes in rank among men. In two separate studies, scientists testing students and prisoners found that

AVOID XENOESTROGENS

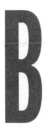

BPA and parabens are just two examples of a class of hormonally active agents called xenoestrogens—chemicals that indirectly provoke the production of, or imitate, estrogen in your body. Found in everything from pesticides and plastic to milk and meats, they can tip the balance and leave you with more estrogen, less T—and a lot more body fat as a result. These man-made estrogens not only disrupt male hormones; they can place you at risk for other health problems. Here are a few other places you'll find xenoestrogens:

YOUR MICROWAVE

Heating up food in the microwave either by placing it in a plastic container or covering it with plastic wrap can cause xenoestrogens within the plastic to leach into your food. Switch to a glass bowl and cover it with a plate if necessary, or use the stove or oven to heat up your food.

YOUR FRIDGE

The average American is exposed to more than 13 different pesticides through food, beverages, and drinking water every day, and most of them are endocrine-disrupting chemicals. The herbicides and synthetic fertilizers that make strawberries, apples, and other fruits and vegetables so big and juicy undermine their healthy benefits. Hormones given to make chickens, cattle, pigs, and turkeys grow plump affect the proper function of our hormonal systems, leading to weight gain and many of the diseases that plague the population. The solution: Buy only organic or naturally grown meats and produce. The more people demand organically raised crops and livestock, the faster prices for these healthy products will come down. If you can't afford organic, then at least wash your produce well to reduce your consumption of xenogenic pesticides.

YOUR GAS STATION

Wash your hands after pumping gas or protect your hands with gloves. Studies show that male gas-station workers have significantly lower levels of testosterone than men who aren't frequently exposed to petrochemicals.

YOUR GARAGE

Sprays and powdered chemicals used to keep pests out of your house or garden also contain xenoestrogens. Use organic weed- and pest-control products instead. Store any nonorganic pest products out of your house in a locked shed to prevent children from coming into contact with them.

testosterone increases in students after graduation and in hostages after they've been released from captivity suggesting a rise in status is responsible. What's more, backing a winner will likely improve your mood, too. Less stress = more T.

T-BOOSTER: COMPETITION

Just as cheering the Red Sox on to victory may elevate testosterone, engaging in a game of pickup basketball or football will likely give you a booster shot of T. Penn State psychology researchers say that competition affects male T-levels in two ways: First, it rises in anticipation of the challenge, and second, it rises in winners and declines in losers.

All-Day Testosterone: Play a team sport after work, but also volunteer for projects at work that involve working as a team and interacting with coworkers. Testosterone studies of collegiate soccer and rugby athletes at Penn State and at Emory University, in Atlanta, suggest that postgame testosterone increases were more strongly associated with team bonding and self-ratings of social connections with teammates than with the outcome of the game. So while playing chess against a computer may give your T a lift, nothing's better than some tribal camaraderie for working up your manly hormones.

T-BOOSTER: WHEY PROTEIN

Make yourself a protein smoothie to boost T and build muscle. More and more research is showing the impact that protein supplements and weight lifting have on strength, muscle building, and testosterone. Researchers in Finland recently found that men who took whey protein before and after a bout of resistance exercise showed a significant change inside their muscles. Specifically, muscle biopsies measured an increase in androgen receptors. These receptors are what testosterone in the blood binds to in order to repair and build muscle. The subjects studied consumed 15 grams of whey protein isolate before and after weight lifting and had muscle biopsies taken during the same intervals. The researchers measured a 25 percent average increase in the ability of the receptors to take up testosterone, and that increase lasted for 48 hours after the men put down the weights.

All-Day Testosterone: The easiest way to trigger the testosterone receptors in your working muscles: Drink a whey protein smoothie. Whey protein is rich in branched-chain amino acids (BCAAs), which have been found to reduce muscle soreness and fatigue after intense exercise. In a study at the University of Connecticut Human Performance Lab, two groups of men were put on a four-week program of intense resistance training. The group that was given amino-acid supplements showed higher testosterone levels and lower markers of muscle damage, and they were able to exercise longer than the group that exercised without protein supplements. (For more T-friendly nutritional supplements, see Chapter 16.)

T-SHIRT CONTEST

Men experience higher testosterone levels when their sexual partners are ovulating, versus other times of the month, according to an experiment at Florida State University. In one study, researchers asked women to wear T-shirts during different phases of their menstrual cycles. Later, they asked men to sniff the T-shirts and then tested their testosterone levels. It turned out that the tees worn by ovulating women elicited the greatest T-boosts in the men.

T-BOOSTER: ERECTIONS

The best noninvasive test for your testosterone level is your "morning wood." If you wake up with an erection, chances are you're doing fine in the T department. A man's testosterone levels are typically highest in the morning; that's because his testicles are busiest producing T while his body is at rest. But research suggests that erections themselves cause a surge in testosterone. In fact, going for long periods without sexual stimulation can actually decrease testosterone levels.

All-Day Testosterone: Have more sex. Not a bad homework assignment, huh? And if that's not possible, then, um, take things into your own hands. A study published in the *Archives of Sexual Behavior* measured blood levels of testosterone in eight men before, during, and after showing them a sexually explicit film. The researchers measured the greatest increase—a 35 percent boost in T—60 to 90 minutes after the film ended.

THE TESTOSTERONE BOMBERS

T-BOMBER: BPA

BPA stands for bisphenol A, a chemical that is used to make polycarbonate plastic and epoxy resins, which are used to line food and beverage cans. Eating foods that have been sitting in plastic containers or cans lined in BPA may reduce your T-levels by exposing you to elevated amounts of estrogenic chemicals that mimic estrogen in your system, causing your body to store more excess body fat. It's these same chemicals that can also interfere with the release of endogenous hormones in your body—a side effect that can decrease your overall testosterone production.

In 2010, Canada declared BPA a toxic substance. The US Food & Drug Administration continues to study BPA; in 2010, it recommended that parents minimize their infants' exposure to the chemical. Even BPA-free plastics may leach estrogenic chemicals, says a study in the journal *Environmental Health Perspectives*.

It gets worse. Even picking up the check could be damaging your testosterone by exposing you to BPA. A Swiss study tested the thermal printer papers used for receipts and discovered that 11 out of 13 contained BPA. (The chemical is a thermal-printing aid.) When subjects touched the paper for 5 seconds, about 1 microgram of BPA found its way onto their fingers—but that number multiplied by about 10 times if their fingers were wet or very greasy. All that BPA stayed on their skin in large concentrations for more than 2 hours afterward. In fact, the researchers concluded that working a cash register for 10 hours could cause a person to be exposed to upwards of 71 micrograms of BPA a day. If you have to handle a receipt, do it quickly and wash your hands as soon as possible, especially before handling foods or placing your fingers anywhere near your mouth.

All-Day Testosterone: Whenever possible, eat all-natural foods or foods that are in certified BPA-free containers. That goes for your water bottle— or whatever you use to drink from—as well. Glass containers and unlined stainless-steel water bottles are the best thing to use, says Heather Patisaul, PhD, who studies hormones and sex differentiation at North Carolina State

University. Never use old or scratched plastic containers, since they can expose you to BPA even more quickly.

How do you know whether a container is made from BPA? The best rule of thumb: Remember Ty Cobb's career batting average (.367), then flip over any product and look for the number on the recycling label. Those with the numbers 3 and 6 contain BPA, and 7 indicates a mix of materials, which means it could contain hazardous ingredients (especially BPA), so steer clear of all three if you want more T. (Numbers 1, 2, and 4 are BPA-free, even if it doesn't say so on the label.)

T-BOMBER: ALCOHOL

Decades of research has shown that drinking too much alcohol hinders testosterone production, as well as sperm count. It's also been shown that excess alcohol consumption speeds up the conversion of testosterone and other androgens responsible for male characteristics into estrogens (the main female sex hormones).

All-Day Testosterone: Try to avoid alcohol for the entire 12-week Testosterone Transformation

THE UPSIDE OF LOWER T

The male sex hormone that helps you to get the girl may change while you're changing diapers—for the benefit of both baby and dad.

Several studies have shown that men with the highest testosterone levels are more likely to find mates and become fathers than men with lower baseline levels of T. But a recent study suggests that testosterone levels decline in married or partnered men who have children compared with men who stay single. The study, led by Northwestern University researchers, also found that men who had a newborn have even lower testosterone than men with older children, and those men who cared for children 3 or more hours a day had lower levels of T than dads not involved in the care of children.

The researchers say interacting with children appears to influence changes in men's hormones, suggesting that men are biologically programmed to be nurturing fathers. The change in hormone levels, they say, may help fathers handle the demands of child-rearing and protect them from certain diseases as they age.

program. But if you like an occasional glass of red wine with dinner, limit yourself to a few glasses each week or less. Same goes for you beer or bourbon drinkers.

T-BOMBER: GROOMING PRODUCTS

Used to be, a can of shaving cream, a stick of deodorant, and a bottle of Old Spice constituted the extent of a man's grooming gear. Not anymore. Today you are using an arsenal of cleansers, creams, lotions, and potions on your scalp and skin to look good and smell clean. Problem is that many of the products in the men's grooming aisles contain parabens, chemicals commonly used as preservatives in cosmetic and pharmaceutical products, such as cleansing gels, makeup, moisturizers and lotions, shampoo, shaving cream, sunscreen, and even toothpaste. Parabens may be great for extending the shelf life of your favorite toiletries, but they can also affect your T-levels, because the chemicals contain estrogen-like properties. One 2004 study published in the *Journal of Applied Toxicology* detected parabens in breast cancer tumors. While the FDA currently doesn't believe that parabens in cosmetics pose a health risk, the agency also doesn't regulate the use of preservatives in cosmetics, so you assume any risk associated with exposure to estrogenic chemicals. In addition to parabens, a common ultraviolet-radiation-blocking chemical used in sunscreens and a variety of cosmetics has been shown to interefere with hormones important to reproduction. According to a recent report in an abstract of *Toxicology*, the UV blocker BP2 (2,2',4,4'-tetrahydroxybenzophenone) decreased testosterone in both cultured human testicular cells and in male mice.

All-Day Testosterone: Don't stop shaving, washing your hair, or using sunscreen, but do try to avoid products containing parabens, BP2, and octinoxate, another chemical UV blocker that may disrupt hormones. Check ingredient listings for words containing "butyl," "ethyl," "methyl," or "propyl." The most common parabens used in cosmetic products are methylparaben, propylparaben, and butylparaben, and you'll usually find more than one type of paraben used or one paraben in combination with other types of preservatives. It won't be easy avoiding parabens—they are found in at least 75 percent of all commercial cosmetic products. But it's easy to spot paraben-free products: Their labels usually boast that benefit boldly. For safer sunscreen, choose a physical UV blocker, such as zinc oxide or titanium dioxide, which lie on top of the skin to prevent UV rays from doing damage.

T-BOMBER:
LOW-FAT DIETS

Fat has undeservedly earned a bad reputation for years. And we're still suffering from the decades-old low-fat food craze, despite the fact that nutrition research has shown how essential fats, especially monounsaturated fats, are for good heart and brain health. Testosterone is another victim of the low-fat misinformation. Eating a very low-fat diet can lead to lower testosterone levels, because healthy dietary fats are critical to the production of testosterone.

All-Day Testosterone: Studies of men have shown that those who eat diets rich in monounsaturated fats like olive oil and the omega-3 fatty acids found in fish had the highest testosterone levels. Some of the best sources for these fats include nuts and seeds, especially flaxseed; fatty cold-water fish like salmon, tuna, and mackerel; avocados; olives; and natural peanut butter.

ALL DAY TESTOSTERONE MADE EASY!

Remember "ALL DAY TEST"—your recipe to maximize testosterone.

+ **A**bstain from alcohol
+ **L**ift heavy and hard
+ **L**imit aerobic activity

+ **D**estress at every opportunity
+ **A**void xenoestrogens
+ **Y**awn less (by sleeping 8 hours nightly)

+ **T**rim belly fat
+ **E**at the right combo of protein, fat, and carbs
+ **S**ex: Have erections often
+ **T**ake T-friendly supplements

TESTOSTERONE THERAPY: SHORTCUT TO MALE VITALITY?

All of your questions about testosterone supplementation answered

CHAPTER

15

Earlier in this book, I cited a study in the *Journal of Clinical Endocrinology* and other research projects, which discovered a curious reduction in the testosterone levels of men in the United States and elsewhere.

One study showed that, on average, a 60 year-old today has about 15 percent less testosterone in his body than a 60-year-old did 20 years earlier.

If T-levels are falling across the board for men, and doctors are so willing to provide testosterone therapy (US doctors alone write 2.5 million T prescriptions a year), one might ask why we shouldn't skip all the hard work in this book and snag a T patch instead?

For answers to this and other common questions about testosterone therapy, I interviewed Darryn S. Willoughby, PhD, an associate professor of exercise/muscle physiology and biochemistry in the Department of Health, Physical Performance, and Recreation at Baylor University in Texas.

Q

SHOULD A MAN CONSIDER TESTOSTERONE THERAPY TO HELP HIM FEEL YOUNGER AND MORE VIGOROUS AS HE AGES?

Darryn S. Willoughby, PhD: That's a subject of great debate. In general, men who have received testosterone supplementation typically report an increase in alertness and well-being, as well as a heightened libido and the ability to gain and sustain an erection. Other benefits that always pique a guy's interest are reports of increases in muscle mass with simultaneous reductions in body fat.

Still, even though testosterone therapy can help reverse the effects of hypogonadism (a medical condition whereby the sex glands produce little or no hormones), it's not clear whether testosterone therapy is that beneficial for older men who are otherwise healthy. Although some men believe that taking testosterone medications may help them feel younger and more vigorous as they age, few clinically controlled research studies have examined testosterone therapy in men who have healthy testosterone levels, with many of these studies producing mixed results.

In light of this, any man considering testosterone therapy should always get a thorough medical screening from his physician first and never attempt to self-administer the drug, due to both medical and legal ramifications. If physician clearance is granted for testosterone therapy, men should weigh the possible benefits against the potential risks with their physician's help.

Q

ARE THE SIGNS AND SYMPTOMS ASSOCIATED WITH AGING ALWAYS DUE TO A NATURAL DECLINE IN TESTOSTERONE?

Dr. Willoughby: Not always. You see, some men can have normal testosterone levels but still display signs and symptoms of aging, while others may have low testosterone (and even be medically considered as hypogonadal) but never display any overt signs or symptoms.

However, for some men, being hypogonadal may result in a number of age-related changes, including an overall loss of energy, as well as changes in sexual function, which may include reduced sexual desire, fewer spontaneous erections, and infertility. There may also be a change in sleep patterns, since low testosterone can cause insomnia and other sleep disturbances.

A number of physical changes can sometimes be associated with hypogonadism as well, including increased body fat, reduced muscle mass and strength, and decreased bone density. Gynecomastia, a condition where testosterone is converted to estrogen in the body, may occur and produce swollen or tender breasts and hair loss. Low testosterone may even produce emotional changes and contribute to a decrease in motivation or self-confidence. There may be feelings of sadness or depression, along with difficulty concentrating or remembering things.

Q

IS THERE A CONNECTION BETWEEN LOW T AND LOW INTEREST IN SEX?

Dr. Willoughby: Yes. Low libido is a common symptom of having low testosterone. But there are many lifestyle issues, particularly nutrition and fitness, that can have a large impact on a man's sex drive, too. For example, being sedentary and having a diet low in essential, unsaturated fatty acids can affect your sex drive. In addition, smoking and drinking can have a detrimental impact on your libido. Still, low testosterone is something a doctor would look to rule out in a patient complaining of low libido or erectile dysfunction, because there is a connection. There are nerves in the brain, which, when stimulated by testosterone, release the compound nitric oxide, which facilitates blood flow into the penis to produce an erection. Testosterone, therefore, is key for firm erections.

Q

WHAT ARE SOME OF THE SIDE EFFECTS AND
RISKS OF TESTOSTERONE THERAPY?

Dr. Willoughby: Some are minor and reversible once taking the drug is ceased. Others are far more severe. Some minor side effects are acne and oily skin, irritability and increased aggression, and sleeping disturbances. More serious side effects can include thinning of the hair or significant hair loss and increased blood pressure.

In addition, testosterone administration can increase prostate size and cause benign prostatic hyperplasia, a non-cancerous enlargement of the gland. It is believed that testosterone supplementation can fuel the growth of any preexisting prostate cancer you may have. Long-term testosterone supplementation can also suppress sperm production and lead to infertility. That's why it's always recommended that physicians screen for prostate cancer with a digital rectal exam and blood levels of prostate-specific antigen before starting testosterone therapy.

Because androgens are associated with increasing the number of red blood cells, a condition known as polycythemia, testosterone therapy has been shown to make the blood thicker and raise blood pressure. Testosterone can also increase cholesterol in your blood, which can elevate your risk for cardiovascular disease. As such, during androgen therapy the physician will typically closely monitor prostate size and the blood levels of hematocrit, cholesterol, and prostate-specific antigen.

Another major concern with testosterone supplementation is misuse of the drug. All the media hype from anabolic-steroid (testosterone) use in the sports world has, in part, increased awareness of the prevalent use of testosterone and the negative side effects associated with it. However, oftentimes athletes and bodybuilders use up to 100 times the medically indicated dosage.

What men need to realize is that testosterone, when given in medically prescribed and indicated dosages by a physician, is normally a safe form of hormone-replacement therapy, particularly for those suffering from either primary hypogonadism or secondary hypogonadism.

A good doctor will do both a biochemical evaluation (to see if a patient truly has testosterone deficiency) and a clinical evaluation (to see if a patient has symptoms that a doctor may feel would improve by replacing testosterone), as well as making sure that they don't have conditions that may be a reason to forgo treatment. For example, if a man has a preexisting condition such as high blood pressure or an enlarged prostate (benign prostate hyperplasia), taking testosterone could magnify the problem.

Q

WHAT ARE THE MOST COMMON CONDITIONS THAT CAN CAUSE A DROP IN A MAN'S TESTOSTERONE LEVELS?

Dr. Willoughby: A head injury, a testicular injury, a vasectomy, and taking certain medications. But the most common condition is age.

As men become older, testosterone levels will lower naturally, due to a decline in normal organ function, particularly those such as the pituitary gland and the hypothalamus in the brain, as well as the Leydig cells in the testes, which release hormones that control the production and release of testosterone.

A brain injury—caused by a stroke, heart attack, or loss of oxygen for long periods of time—also may result in lowered testosterone levels. This is due to the fact that oxygen deprivation may cause damage to the pituitary gland and the hypothalamus, both which are critical in testosterone production.

A testicular injury can also affect testosterone production due to damage of the Leydig cells within the testes.

Contrary to what most men believe to be the case, vasectomies don't always result in lower testosterone levels. However, in some cases, a vasectomy can result in an autoimmune disorder in which your body begins to develop antibodies against testicular tissue. Those same antibodies invariably destroy the Leydig cells, thereby reducing testosterone production.

ARE THERE MEDICATIONS THAT REDUCE A MAN'S T-LEVELS, AND WHAT EXACTLY ARE THEY DOING TO CAUSE THAT EFFECT?

Dr. Willoughby: There are a number of classifications of medications that can reduce testosterone, such as antihypertensive drugs (Inderal, Clonidine, Reserpine, Lasix, etc.), antidepressants (such as selective serotonin reuptake inhibitors, or SSRIs), tricyclics, monoamine oxidase inhibitors, (MAOIs), tranquilizers (Haldol, Thorazine, Zyprexa, Seroquel, etc.), and anticholinergics (Benadryl, Donnatal, Pro-Banthine, Cogentin, etc.).

All of these classifications of drugs can increase or decrease the levels of various hormones in the body, which can suppress the body's production and release of testosterone by affecting the hypothalamus in the brain. They also have the ability to damage the nervous, vascular, and endocrine systems—from inhibiting the release of certain neurotransmitters to increasing fluid loss and reducing blood pressure, which can also lower testosterone production.

Q

IF A MAN IS A CANDIDATE FOR TESTOSTERONE REPLACEMENT, WHAT ARE SOME OF THE MEDICAL CHOICES AVAILABLE?

Dr. Willoughby: Testosterone therapy can involve the injection of testosterone esters (such as testosterone cypionate or testosterone enanthate), transdermal skin patches (Androderm), implants under the skin, oral tablets (such as Andriol), topical gels (AndroGel, Testogel and Testim), and topical creams (such as AndroForte).

Q
HOW OFTEN DO THEY HAVE TO BE TAKEN TO BE EFFECTIVE?

Dr. Willoughby: It depends on what form your doctor decides is right for you. Testosterone injections are typically given once weekly, although the other forms of testosterone therapy mentioned earlier need to be taken daily. The reason why is because testosterone injections are usually more effective, since the concentration of the dose is usually higher and the drug is directly injected. The other forms of testosterone delivery are also effective, but not as much, because the concentration of the dose is less and the route of delivery is less direct than with injections.

If you're wondering how long a typical course of testosterone therapy lasts, it can range from several weeks to several months. That decision is usually based on various clinical evaluations, such as prostate screening and blood testing for red-blood-cell counts and cholesterol.

Q
WHAT ABOUT ALL THOSE NATURAL NUTRITIONAL SUPPLEMENTS THAT SUPPOSEDLY INCREASE TESTOSTERONE? DO THEY WORK?

Dr. Willoughby: There's no question the nutritional-supplement market is flooded with products that can be taken orally that are alleged "testosterone boosters." Several of these natural supplements may be beneficial in elevating testosterone based on results from clinically controlled scientific studies. However, it's important to understand that the Food and Drug Administration has no role in testing and evaluating the effectiveness and safety parameters of these products. Because of that, no clinical dosage of these products has been established, so how much to take can be a risky guessing game. Furthermore, if you're considering taking any "natural testosterone-boosting" product, it's imperative that you discuss it first with your physician. Why? Because if it happens to be effective, you may be at risk for the same types of side effects and medical concerns related to doctor-prescribed testosterone therapy.

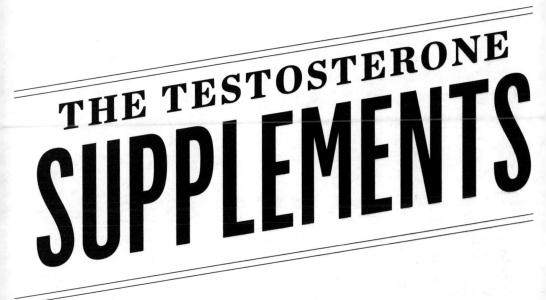

THE TESTOSTERONE SUPPLEMENTS

Nutritional add-ons that may optimize muscle growth

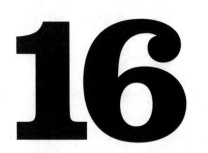

CHAPTER

16

SUP·PLE·MENT

(n.): **something that completes or makes an addition.**

That's a key definition, because it's important to recognize that nowhere in it will you find the words "magic bullet" or "the answer."

By definition, a supplement is an adjunct, a helper, a supporter of something larger, but not an essential element. I bring this up because the advertisements for many so-called T-raising, muscle-building supplements in magazines and online would have you believe that swallowing this product or that will help you get massive benefits instantly. Baloney. And you know it. Still, hundreds of thousands of men spend big money on supplements believing they are a shortcut and a substitute for eating right and exercising hard.

The single biggest mistake men make when it comes to taking supplements isn't taking the wrong types or the ones that don't work at all, but taking them in lieu of watching what they eat, working out the right way, and following healthy lifestyle habits. If that's you, then we have NEWS for you. You won't reach your goals by searching for shortcuts through supplements. Nutritionals can help, but only after you've built a strong foundation with the crucial building blocks of muscle. They are, in order of importance:

→ **N**utrition
→ **E**xercise
→ **W**ay of Life
→ **S**upplements

Nutrition and exercise really run neck and neck in importance. But notice what's at the very bottom: supplements.

To get your money's worth from nutritional supplements, you need the right diet, the right exercise plan, and healthy lifestyle habits in place first. Otherwise those powders and pills will be the most expensive and useless (and unsatisfying, from your taste buds' perspective) stuff you ever paid for.

That said, there's a place for supplements in the Testosterone Transformation program. There's significant scientific evidence that taking the right mix of certain nutritional supplements can accelerate and enhance the benefits of all your NEW efforts by helping your body train harder, recuperate faster, preserve lean muscle, and utilize more stored fat as fuel.

Below is a list of seven superior T-friendly supplements. Some are safe and natural alternatives that encourage your body to release more testosterone, while others work to preserve all of the new lean muscle you've built as a result of all that extra T.

A few things you won't find in this grouping include pro-hormone products, estrogen blockers, or any type of supplement that binds to receptors or manipulates your hormone levels in an unnatural way.

There are only two rules we recommend following. One: Always check with your doctor before considering any supplements you might not be as familiar with. Two, even if you get a green light to try everything in this chapter, don't try all of these supplements at once. Everyone's chemistry is different, and yours might make significant gains with a certain supplement yet never experience any noticeable difference using another type of supplement. So test them out individually. It will save you money, time, and disappointment in the long run.

So as tempting as it might be to start popping supplements, we recommend that you jump into the Testosterone Transformation program without supplements to start. (However, if you currently take a multivitamin or other supplements, you can continue.) Trust us when we say you will see and feel the difference from the diet, workout, and lifestyle changes alone. But if you take supplements at the start of this program, you'll never be absolutely certain what's really having the greatest effect on your physique.

Once you're used to the plan—and have experienced the strength, size, and muscular changes that come from the Testosterone Transformation way of exercising and eating—then you can comfortably try experimenting with two or three supplements at a time for one month. After that, you can begin adding one or two other supplements, depending on your budget. If you do it this way, you'll be more likely to identify what is truly working for you—and what may be too costly compared with the return you're getting on your exercise investment.

THE T-FRIENDLY SUPPLEMENTS

1 MULTIVITAMIN

Your body's ability to produce testosterone and other anabolic hormones that influence muscular growth depends on many factors, but the most important— yet often overlooked—is having nutritional balance.

If you're lacking in any nutrient because of a poor or imbalanced diet, it's like trying to score a touchdown without a running back. Every essential vitamin and mineral is like a player on your body's team, all of whom must come together to win the game.

When they're all in play, your odds of winning are high—but, more important, it also takes less effort to play well. For your body, having every nutrient means it can run at maximum efficiency—and that means being more efficient at handling all of the day-to-day metabolic chores it's responsible for, including producing plenty of testosterone. Unfortunately, most men don't get optimum amounts of crucial vitamins from their diets alone. That's why a good multivitamin is the least expensive insurance policy you'll ever buy.

Choose a multi that has 100 percent of the recommended daily allowance (RDA) of each vitamin and mineral, especially vitamins C and E, calcium, magnesium, vitamin D, and omega-3 fatty acids (these are the nutrients that most men tend to be deficient in).

Best T Time: Take your multi with breakfast. Why? It's easier to digest and process a multi when it's consumed with a whole-food meal, and you'll give your body everything it needs at the beginning of the day.

2 WHEY AND CASEIN PROTEIN

Protein is so important to building muscle and increasing testosterone that not only does it have its own chapter (see Chapter 5), but this book even spells out the best time to consume it (see page 40). Remember, protein is also a fat burner. According to a study by British researchers, people who increased the percentage of calories from protein in their meals burned 71 more calories per day than people on low-protein diets. We recommend whey and casein protein powder supplements mixed in a smoothie, for instance, because they offer an easy way to get quality protein that contains essential amino acids for building muscle and burning fat. Combining both types of protein supplements offers a dual-action effect. Whey is absorbed quickly, so it feeds your muscles immediately; casein is more slowly digested, allowing it to provide muscle-building nutrients for a longer period.

Beyond that, protein powders make life easier on the Testosterone Transformation program. Sometimes it's difficult to consume our recommended 1 gram of protein per pound of body weight per day from meat and dairy products alone. Protein supplements are simple to measure and convenient to consume, especially as before-and-after workout snacks. To avoid lumpy protein drinks, get yourself a good blender, one with at least 400 watts of ice-chopping power under the hood. Here are some other ways to use protein powder supplements:

▶ Stir into cottage cheese or oatmeal.

▶ Mix whey protein powder into pancake or waffle batter.

▶ Add it to oat flour when baking muffins and cakes.

3 CREATINE

Hundreds of studies have revealed that creatine has the ability to increase muscle strength, power, and size. One of its jobs is helping draw more water into your muscle cells, leaving them looking fuller, larger, and harder. When taken before and after workouts, that surge can help drive certain key nutrients and fluids straight into your muscles, which can help speed up their recovery after you hit them hard.

This super-supplement is actually a naturally occurring compound made primarily by the liver by combining the amino acids glycine, arginine, and methionine. You can also find it in meat and fish. But you can get only 1 gram of creatine from a whole pound of meat, so unless you prefer throwing back an entire cow, the most efficient source is a powdered supplement.

Creatine products go by many names, the most common being creatine monohydrate. Some of the newer versions that seem to cause less of a bloated feeling in the stomach—a symptom that some men experience on creatine monohydrate—include creatine-alpha-ketoglutarate, creatine ethyl ester, creatine gluconate, and creatine methyl ester.

Creatine is important for many reasons. It has been shown to boost the intracellular pool of phosphocreatine within your skeletal muscle, which allows your muscles to regenerate adenosine triphosphate (ATP) more rapidly; ATP is the energy source that allows your muscles to contract. As you work out, muscle contractions deplete ATP reserves, so having more ATP gives your muscles more fuel to burn, allowing them to work out harder and longer with less fatigue. Because of this effect, most men experience a performance increase in their strength-training workouts of 5 to 10 percent on average. Research also has shown that creatine aids in protein synthesis, decreases protein breakdown, and boosts levels of certain key anabolic hormones. According to a study published in the *International Journal of Sport Nutrition and Exercise Metabolism*, supplementing with creatine during resistance-exercise training increased the concentration of intramuscular insulin-like growth factor 1 (a key hormone that plays a major role in helping your body build muscle) in men.

Best T Time: Take 3 to 5 grams in a protein shake before and after you exercise, but don't exceed 10 grams daily. On non-training days, take only 3 to 5 grams at breakfast time, preferably with grape juice or in a protein shake. The reason: Eating either a large amount of glucose (roughly 80 to 100 grams) or a carbohydrate/protein mixture (50 to 80 grams of carbs, 20 to 40 grams of protein) has been shown to raise insulin, which enhances your muscles' ability to uptake creatine into their cells.

4 Omega-3 (EPA and DHA)

We include fish oil in this list because it is so important to the healthy functioning of your body. Fish oil is the only dietary supplement consistently shown in clinical trials to prevent heart-attack death by stabilizing the heart's electrical system. It's known to lower blood pressure and triglycerides and slow the buildup of arterial plaque. Omega-3s are found in fatty fish like salmon, tuna, and mackerel, but many people find that fish oil supplements are more convenient than cooking fish two or three times a week. Besides its anti-inflammatory properties, omega-3s have mood-elevating effects. They have been shown to relieve depression as effectively as antidepressant medications and reduce the risk of cognitive decline.

Best T time: Take 1,000 milligrams of a supplement containing the omega-3s EPA and DHA combined daily.

5 BCAAs

BCAA stands for "branched-chain amino acid," and these three amino acids— leucine, isoleucine, and valine—are critical to muscle growth.

Collectively, these important amino acids are responsible for repairing and building muscle tissue by promoting muscle-protein synthesis. In addition, they work together to give you more energy as you exercise, to lower your levels of cortisol (the catabolic hormone that impedes the release of testosterone and causes muscles to break down), and to minimize delayed-onset muscle soreness—the syndrome that occurs 24 to 48 hours after intensive exercise that can inhibit your performance during future workouts.

Leucine—the most essential of the three—even goes a step further to protect your T-built physique by boosting the release of the anabolic hormone insulin, which aids in protein synthesis and also accelerates nutrients such as glucose and amino acids into your muscle cells. That window of opportunity is most critical immediately after you exercise, when your muscles desperately need to replenish what they've lost through exercise and to begin the process of repairing themselves.

One study, performed at the College of Charleston's Department of Health and Human Performance, examined the effects of BCAA supplementation on men during periods of high-intensity resistance training. After four weeks, subjects who took BCAAs had a significantly higher amount of serum testosterone and a significantly lower amount of cortisol, suggesting that short-term amino acid supplementation (high in BCAAs) may have a net anabolic hormonal effect and increase performance while decreasing muscle break-down and cell damage. In short, BCAA supplementation can speed up recovery and lower your risk of injury.

When choosing a BCAA supplement, look for a blend that offers a 2:1:1 ratio of leucine, isoleucine, and valine. If a serving is 5 grams, then you'll get 2.5 grams of leucine, 1.25 grams of isoleucine, and 1.25 grams of valine.
Best T Time: Take 5 to 10 grams on an empty stomach in the morning, 5 to 10 grams within the 30 minutes before your workout, and 5 to 10 grams immediately after your workout.

6 GLUTAMINE

Glutamine might be the most prevalent naturally occurring amino acid in your body, but that doesn't mean investing in it in supplement form is a waste of money. Glutamine is one of the best muscle-building supplements you can take for several reasons: It boosts your immune system, elevates your growth-hormone levels, and increases the number of calories and fat you expend as you exercise, and even at rest. The mighty amino acid also helps in the production of bicarbonate, which works to reduce the lactic acid left inside your muscles after intense exercise so your muscles feel less sore and fatigued afterward. The less discomfort your muscles feel, the harder and longer you'll be able to push them in future workouts.

Glutamine assists in transporting glycogen into your muscle cells—glycogen that in turn draws more water into your muscle cells so they stay hydrated, work more efficiently, and appear larger and fuller. But some experts say that the biggest advantage to maintaining a high level of glutamine is that it helps to regulate protein synthesis, allowing your body to convert protein into muscle tissue more quickly.

Here's the irony: Although your body makes glutamine, this muscle aid pulls other amino acids from your body—specifically from your muscles! By adding glutamine into your nutritional regime, your muscles are spared from being cannibalized, so they can grow even bigger.

Best T Time: Take 5 to 10 grams with your breakfast, 5 to 10 grams right before your workout, 5 to 10 grams immediately after your workout, and 5 to 10 grams right before bedtime. You can mix it in your beverages, and it's fine to mix with creatine and BCAAs in your protein shakes.

7 ZMA

ZMA—a combination of zinc, magnesium aspartate, and vitamin B6—works in your favor in several key ways, including giving you a natural boost in IGF-1 (insulin-like growth factor 1), a natural protein with anabolic effects.

First and foremost, ZMA supplementation ensures that you're never deficient in zinc, a critical mineral that gets gobbled up whenever you perform intense exercise. The problem: suffering from a zinc deficiency can affect your pituitary gland's ability to release certain hormones that stimulate testosterone production. Zinc is also crucial when it comes to protein synthesis, so by getting enough through diet and supplements, you speed up your body's ability to make the muscle.

Magnesium, on the other hand, is an essential mineral that also has been shown to give T-levels a boost. More important, it has been shown to protect against heart disease and Type 2 diabetes. Researchers believe that 56 percent of the population consumes inadequate amounts of this mineral. In addition, magnesium can help enhance the quality of sleep you're already getting.

Best T Time: Pick a product that has a ratio of 30 milligrams of zinc, 450 milligrams of magnesium, and 10 milligrams of vitamin B6. Take it 30 to 60 minutes before bedtime on an empty stomach—this allows your body to absorb the combination much faster. If you do have a late-night snack, make sure you don't ingest any calcium, as this mineral can block ZMA absorption.

8 CAFFEINE

This central-nervous-system stimulant doesn't have a direct effect on your T-levels. Instead, caffeine's longtime role as an exercise supplement is more like insurance that you'll stay alert and focused enough when working out.

Taking caffeine may also help your muscles function more efficiently during exercise. A recent study in Italy examined the muscle-fiber conduction velocity in male subjects after giving them caffeine and having them perform biceps curls. The result: Muscle-fiber conduction velocity was 8.7 percent higher in subjects who had consumed caffeine, which means that it may actually improve your neuromuscular function, particularly during intense dynamic exercise.

Caffeine provides a fat-loss edge. When taken at the right time—and in the right quantity—caffeine can cause your body to use a greater percentage of stored fat (instead of muscle glycogen) as you exercise, which can leave you leaner-looking in the long run with less effort.

Best T Time: Try drinking one or two cups of coffee, or an energy drink containing around 200 milligrams of caffeine, immediately before exercise. However, if you typically exercise in the evenings and find that caffeine prevents you from getting the recommended daily amount of T-boosting sleep, then either try working out earlier or skip this one altogether.

BONUS CHAPTER

THE MIXED MARTIAL ARTS
WORKOUT

When you're ready, here's a fast, effective (and tough) way to incinerate fat

CHAPTER

17

Mixed martial arts fighters are among the fittest professional athletes on the planet. The moment any MMA fighter steps into the cage, ring, or Octagon and begins swinging, there's no question his body is pumping out testosterone about as intensely as his fists and feet are pummeling his opponent. However, boosting testosterone levels is never the first priority for a fighter preparing for a bout. Most of the time, it's about helping the athlete make weight without losing the power and stamina he's built up during months of training.

The bonus workout on the following pages has that goal in mind for you, too: losing weight while keeping your muscle. It will help you fry those last stubborn pounds while maintaining the muscle, strength, and athletic ability you've built during these past 12 weeks on the Testosterone Transformation Workout.

Meet Kelly Tekin: This MMA Fighter Workout was created by Kelly Tekin, MS, a nationally ranked bodybuilder, former professional women's soccer player for Germany, and renowned strength-and-conditioning coach. She is the coach behind some of the world's fittest MMA fighters, including top-ranked light heavyweight champ Jon "Bones" Jones, highly decorated Muay Thai kickboxer James "the Hammer" McSweeney, and former UFC light heavyweight champion Rashad Evans.

You're going to love this workout. It requires no special equipment, so you can do it just about anywhere. And it is plenty challenging. In fact, it's not for everyone.

"Although this routine will definitely increase your testosterone levels, it's not for a beginner lifter," says Tekin. You should have a good six months of weight training under your belt before giving it a try. We recommend you perform the 12-week Testosterone Transformation Workout twice through or the Maximum Strength Advanced Workout before jumping into the ring with Kelly.

But when you're ready, have at it:

The Time-Saving, T-Boosting, MMA-Style Workout from Hell

Strength training is just one element in a mixed martial artist's training program. Other aspects, like sparring, ground work, technique training, and road work, compete for the athlete's time, so strength training needs to be efficient and simple—no cable or weight-stack machines to get in the way. Besides, few MMA workout facilities have that kind of equipment. Tekin's routine requires only a barbell, a flat bench, a medicine ball, and a few dumbbells.

Her program is divided into two full-body workouts, each made up of eight exercises. You will perform them at a fast tempo that raises your heart rate to help burn body fat. These workouts are so effective that you'll need to exercise only two or three times per week.

THE MIXED MARTIAL ARTS WORKOUT

DAY 1

For this workout, you'll perform all sets of an exercise before moving on to the next exercise. Rest for 30 to 45 seconds between each set, and for 90 to 120 seconds between exercises. Before moving to the Day Two workout, wait 48 hours for your muscles to recover.

How to warm up before the workout: Pedal a stationary cycle or bicycle at a slow pace for 30 seconds, then increase the resistance significantly (or switch to a lower gear) and pedal fast for 30 seconds. Repeat this pattern 5 to 8 times over the course of 5 to 8 minutes.

Exercise	REPS	SETS
SQUAT (3 FOOT POSITIONS)	15 total (5+5+5)	4
ROMANIAN DEADLIFT	5	5
BENT-OVER BARBELL ROW (underhand grip)	15 total (5+5+5)	4
3-2-1 BENCH PRESS	6	4
FRONT-AND-BACK BARBELL SHOULDER PRESS	20 total (10+10)	4
STANDING TRICEPS EXTENSION	8	4
ALTERNATING HAMMER CURL	8 with each arm	1
MEDICINE-BALL POWER-UP	10	3

(EXERCISE DESCRIPTIONS FOLLOW ON PAGE 282.)

SQUAT

REPS 15 (THREE FOOT POSITIONS; 5+5+5)   **SETS** 4

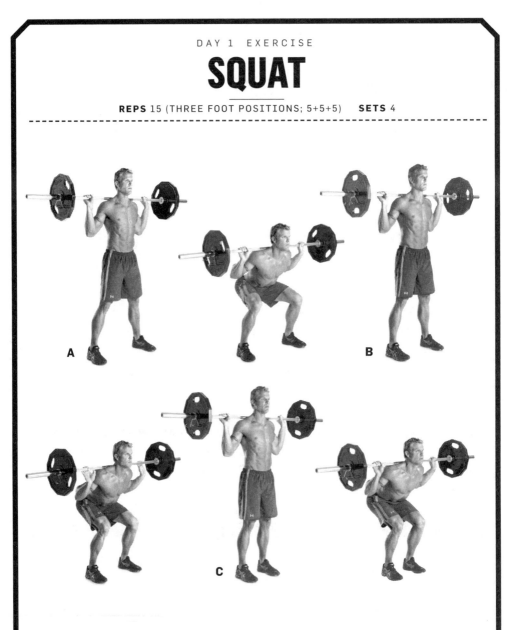

START POSITION

➡ Rest a barbell across the back of your shoulders and grab the bar with an overhand grip, hands slightly more than shoulder-width apart. Space your feet more than shoulder-width apart.

THE MOVE: (A) Keeping your back straight, squat down until your thighs are parallel to the floor. Press yourself back up into a standing position, stopping just short of locking your knees. Repeat this a total of 5 times.

(B) Immediately bring your feet in closer so they're shoulder-width apart and do 5 more reps.

(C) Immediately bring your feet in even closer so that they're about hip-width apart and repeat the exercise for a final 5 reps.

ROMANIAN DEADLIFT

REPS 5 **SETS** 5

- -

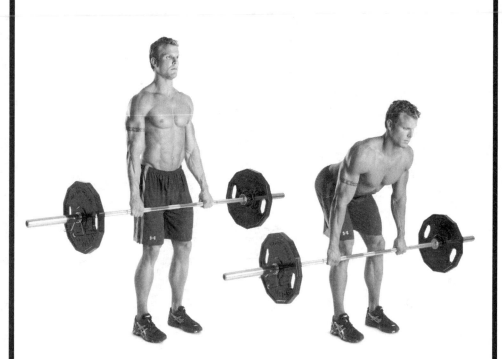

START POSITION

➜ Stand holding a barbell with an overhand grip, arms hanging down in front of your legs. Your feet should be shoulder-width apart, knees slightly bent.

THE MOVE: With your back arched and your chest held high, push your hips back, bend your knees, and lower the barbell to just below your knees—your head and chest should stay up as you go. Push yourself back up into the starting position by pressing through your heels and straightening your legs. Keep the bar as close to your body as possible. Repeat.

BENT-OVER BARBELL ROW
(Underhand Grip)

REPS 15 TOTAL (5+5+5)   **SETS** 4

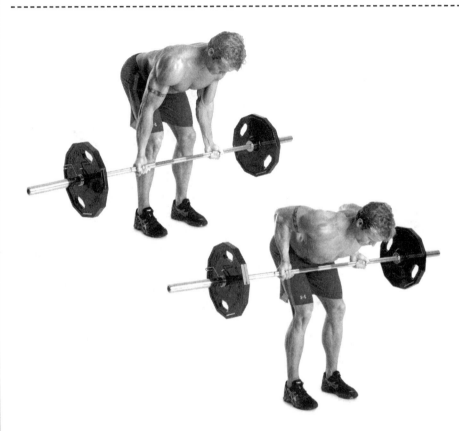

START POSITION

➜ Stand behind a barbell with your feet shoulder-width apart. Bend at the waist and grab the bar with your palms facing forward, hands slightly wider than shoulder-width apart. Lift the barbell off the floor and position your torso so it's slightly above parallel to the floor. (Your arms should hang straight below you.)

THE MOVE: Keeping your back flat and your legs slightly bent, quickly pull the bar up until it touches your midsection right between your lower chest and your belly button. Slowly lower it until your arms are straight. That's 1 rep. Repeat 5 times.

Without resting, add 5 to 20 pounds (depending on your strength level) to the barbell and repeat for 5 more reps.

Finish the exercise by increasing the weight by another 5 to 20 pounds (depending on your strength level) and repeat for 5 reps.

3-2-1 BENCH PRESS

REPS 6   **SETS** 4

START POSITION

➜ Lie face up on an exercise bench with knees bent, feet flat on floor. Grab a barbell with an overhand grip, hands slightly wider than shoulder-width apart. Lift the bar off the rack and hold it directly above your chest, arms straight and perpendicular to the floor.

THE MOVE: Slowly lower the bar to your chest—take a full 3 seconds to lower it. Pause for 2 seconds at the bottom of the move. Now forcefully push the bar back up above your chest until your arms are straight, elbows unlocked. Immediately repeat the exercise—do not rest at the top of the move.

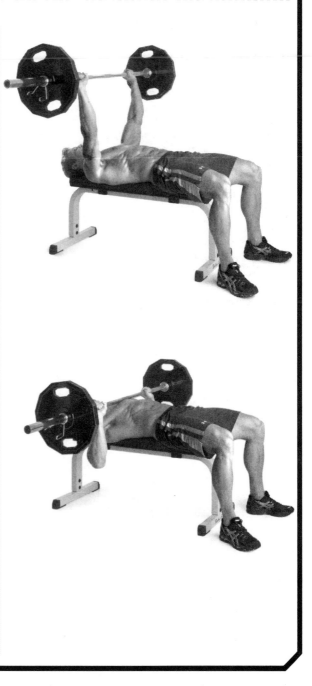

★ TRAINER'S TIP

Using this 3-2-1 cadence engages your muscles through three types of contractions: eccentric (as you lower the weight slowly), isometric (when you pause for 2 seconds), and concentric (as you push the weight up explosively). Each type of contraction utilizes different arrangements of muscle fibers within the same muscle group, so you exhaust them more thoroughly.

FRONT-AND-BACK BARBELL SHOULDER PRESS

REPS 20 TOTAL (10+10)   **SETS** 4

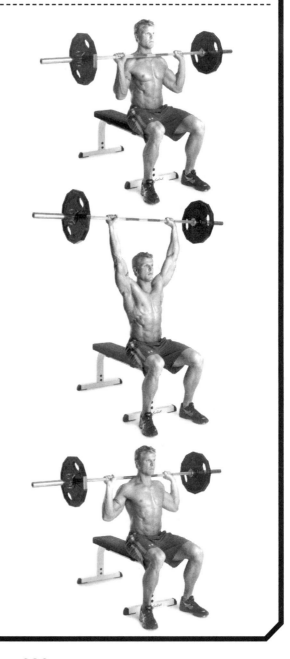

START POSITION

➡ Sit on a bench facing a barbell rack with your feet flat on the floor. Grab the bar in front of you with your hands slightly more than shoulder-width apart and rest it just across the top of your chest.

THE MOVE: Press the weight up above your head until your arms are straight, elbows unlocked. Pause, then lower the bar to your chest. Repeat for 10 reps. Press the weight back above you, then lower it—this time down to the back of your neck, as if you were placing the bar across your shoulders to perform a squat. Press the weight back up and repeat for 10 reps.

STANDING TRICEPS EXTENSION

REPS 8 **SETS** 4

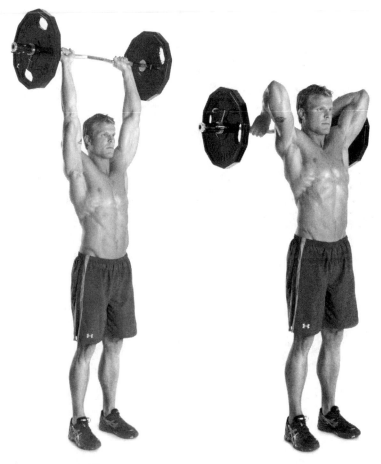

START POSITION

➜ Grab a barbell (or E-Z curl bar) with an overhand grip and your hands shoulder-width or less apart. Stand straight with your feet hip-width apart. Press the bar over your head until your arms are fully extended, palms facing forward.

THE MOVE: Keeping your upper arms close to your head and your elbows in, slowly bend your arms to lower the bar behind your head for a five count. (Only your forearms should move—your upper arms should stay stationary throughout the movement.) Once your forearms touch your biceps, immediately raise the weight back up over your head as quickly as possible until your arms are straight, and repeat without pausing at the top.

ALTERNATING HAMMER CURL

REPS 8 WITH EACH ARM   **SETS** 1

To do this exercise, you'll need a rack of various-size dumbbells
that let you work your way down in weight.

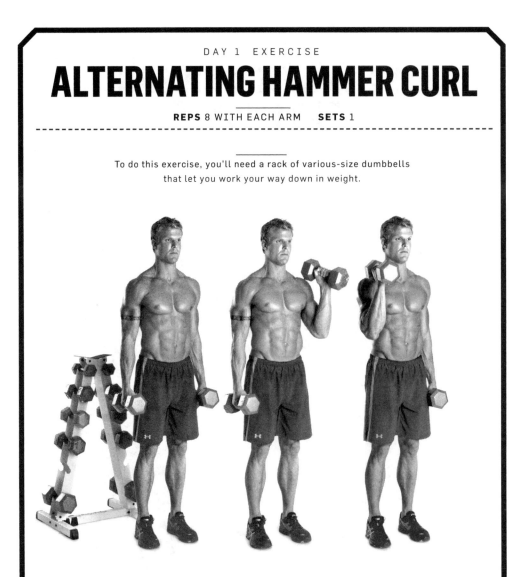

START POSITION

➡ Choose a pair of dumbbells you can barely curl for 8 full repetitions. Stand straight with a
dumbbell in each hand, arms down at your sides, and palms facing your thighs.

THE MOVE: Keeping your back straight, slowly curl the dumbbell in your left hand toward your
left shoulder, keeping your wrist from turning as you go. Your thumb should be pointing toward your
shoulder at the top of the move. Lower the weight until your arm is straight and repeat, this time with
your right arm. Alternate from left to right and do 8 reps with each arm, for a total of 16 reps.

Immediately grab a pair of dumbbells 5 to 10 pounds lighter than the pair you just used and
repeat the exercise for another 16 reps. For example, if you were curling 45-pound dumbbells, grab
a pair of either 35- or 40-pound dumbbells. Continue to work down the rack, repeating the exercise
until you finish with either the 15- or 20-pound dumbbells.

MEDICINE-BALL POWER-UP

REPS 10   **SETS** 3

For this exercise, you'll need a medicine ball and a mat or other soft surface.

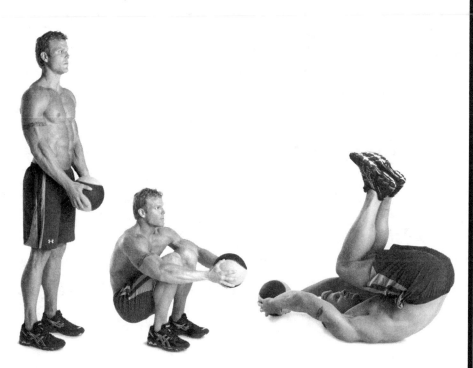

START POSITION

➜ Stand straight with your feet about 6 inches apart. Hold a medicine ball with both hands in front of your waist.

THE MOVE: Squat down as deep as you can so that the backs of your thighs touch your calves, and try to touch your butt to the floor. Continue to roll backward and draw your knees up toward the sides of your head as you simultaneously sweep your arms back to touch the ball on the floor right behind your head. At the end, you should be curled up into a ball, resting only on your upper back and shoulders.

Reverse the motion, but instead of returning to a standing position, jump up as high as you can, raising the ball over your head. Land softly and immediately repeat the exercise so that the set is one continuous movement.

THE MIXED MARTIAL ARTS WORKOUT

DAY 2

For this workout, you'll perform all eight of the exercises as a circuit, that is, back-to-back with no rest between exercises. So, for example, you will complete one set of the bent-over barbell row and then move immediately into the straight-leg deadlift, and so on. Note: You will use a lighter weight load to allow you to complete all sets of the eight exercises without resting.

Once you've finished the circuit, you'll rest for 60 to 120 seconds, then immediately perform the eight-move cycle once again. Continue this way until you've completed five full circuits. The rest rules for Day One apply to Day Two—wait at least 48 hours between workouts, but no more than 72 hours, to allow your muscles an adequate time to repair and recover.

How to warm up before the workout: Jog for 30 seconds, then sprint for 30 seconds. Repeat this pattern five to eight times.

EXERCISE	REPS	SETS
BENT-OVER BARBELL ROW (underhand grip)	10	5
STRAIGHT-LEG DEADLIFT	10	5
HANG CLEAN	10	5
FRONT SQUAT	10	5
PUSH PRESS	10	5
SQUAT	10	5
ALTERNATING FORWARD LUNGE	10 total (5 reps each leg)	5
BARBELL JUMP SQUAT	10	5

BENT-OVER BARBELL ROW
(Underhand Grip)

REPS 10   **SETS** 5

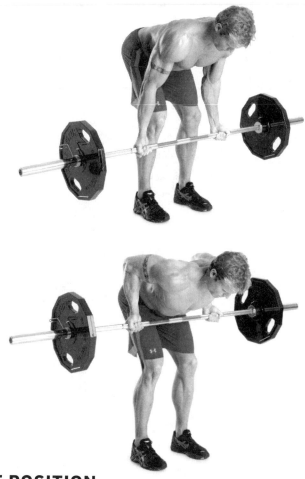

START POSITION

→ Stand behind a barbell with your feet shoulder-width apart. Bend at the waist and grab the bar with your palms facing forward, hands slightly wider than shoulder-width apart. Lift the barbell off the floor and position your torso so it's slightly above parallel to the floor. (Your arms should hang straight below you.)

THE MOVE: Keeping your back flat and your legs slightly bent, quickly pull the bar up until it touches your midsection between your lower chest and belly button. Slowly lower it back down until your arms are straight, and repeat.

STRAIGHT-LEG DEADLIFT

REPS 10   **SETS** 5

START POSITION

→ Stand holding a barbell with an overhand grip—arms hanging down in front of your legs. Your feet should be shoulder-width apart, knees slightly bent.

THE MOVE: Bend at the hips and lower your torso until it's parallel to the floor. Raise yourself back to the starting position and repeat.

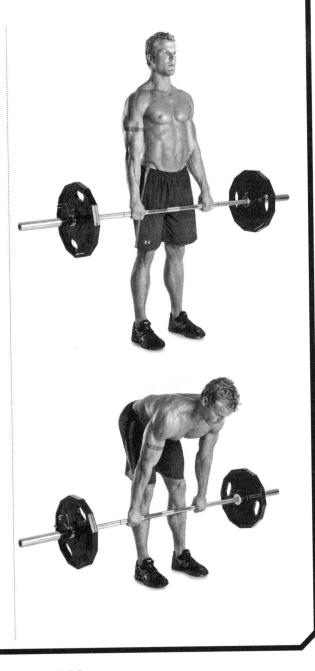

HANG CLEAN

REPS 10   **SETS** 5

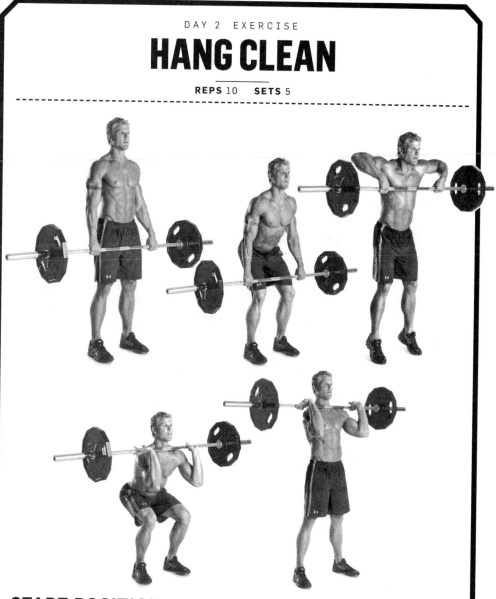

START POSITION

➜ Stand straight, holding a barbell with an overhand grip (hands shoulder-width apart), and let your arms hang straight so the bar rests in front of your thighs.

THE MOVE: Keeping your midsection tight, bend your knees and push your hips back (as if you're getting ready to jump straight up) until the bar reaches the middle of your thighs. Next, in one continuous motion, shrug your shoulders as you bend your elbows, rise up on your toes, and forcefully pull the bar upward to your chest. Once the bar reaches chest height, bend your knees and quickly rotate your forearms underneath the bar to catch it on the front of your shoulders. (You should be in a squat position with your elbows high and out in front of you when you catch the bar.) Stand up, then return the weight to the start position and repeat.

FRONT SQUAT

REPS 10 **SETS** 5

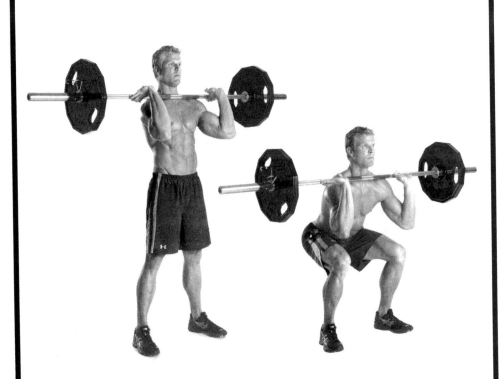

START POSITION

➔ Grab a barbell with an overhand grip slightly more than shoulder-width apart. Raise your elbows up in front of you so that your upper arms are parallel to the floor. Allow the bar to roll back so that it's resting on the front of your shoulders.

THE MOVE: Keeping your torso straight, slowly bend your knees and squat down until your thighs are parallel to the floor. Pause, then push yourself up until your legs are straight—knees unlocked— and repeat. Keep your weight on your heels, not your toes, throughout the movement. If your weight is distributed correctly, you should be able to wiggle your toes at any moment during the lift.

PUSH PRESS

REPS 10   **SETS** 5

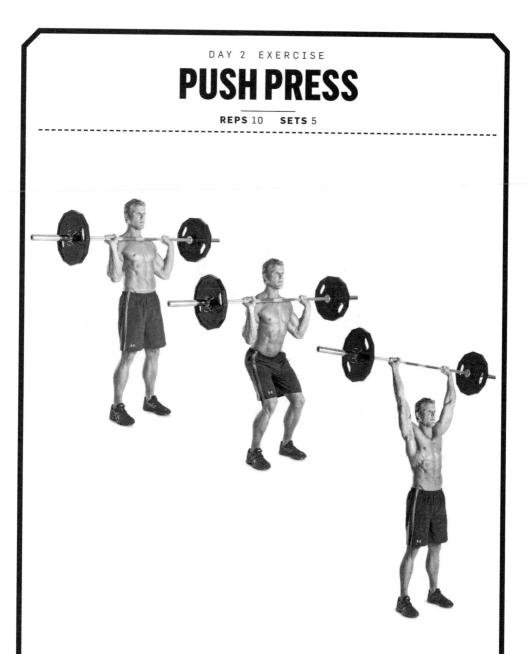

START POSITION

➔ Grab a barbell with an overhand grip that's just beyond shoulder-width and hold it on your upper chest at shoulder level.

THE MOVE: Lift your chest high by taking a deep breath, then tighten your core muscles—they should remain tight throughout the entire exercise. Bend your knees slightly so that you lower yourself down about a foot, then forcefully push through your heels as you quickly stand up and press the bar over your head until your arms are straight. Lower the bar back to your upper chest and repeat.

SQUAT

REPS 10   **SETS** 5

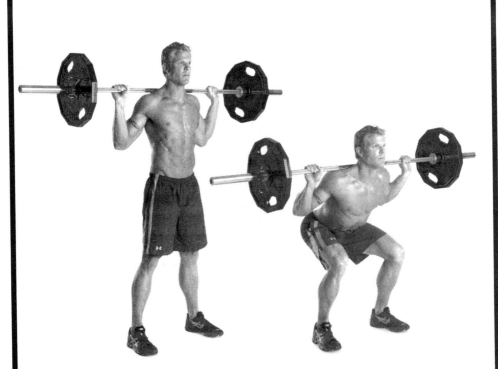

START POSITION

➡ Rest a barbell across the back of your shoulders, holding the bar with an overhand grip, hands slightly more than shoulder-width apart. Space your feet shoulder-width apart.

THE MOVE: Keeping your back straight, push your hips back and lower your body until your thighs are parallel to the floor. Pause, then reverse the movement by driving your heels into the floor to stand up. Stop just short of locking your knees. Repeat.

ALTERNATING FORWARD LUNGE

REPS 10   **SETS** 5

START POSITION

➡ Place a barbell across your upper back and grab the bar with an overhand grip, hands more than shoulder-width apart. Stand with your feet shoulder-width apart.

THE MOVE: Step forward with your left foot, bending your left knee until your left thigh is parallel to the floor, keeping your back as straight as possible. Quickly push yourself back into a standing position and repeat the exercise, this time stepping forward with your right foot. Alternate legs (5 reps each) for a total of 10 reps.

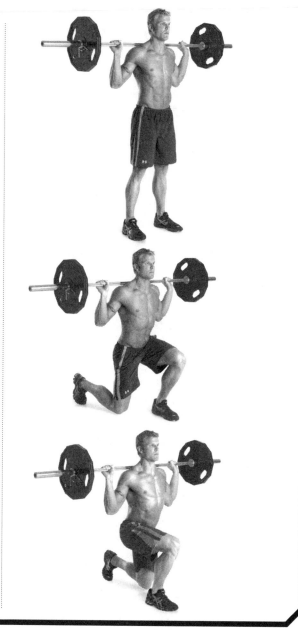

BARBELL JUMP SQUAT

REPS 10   **SETS** 5

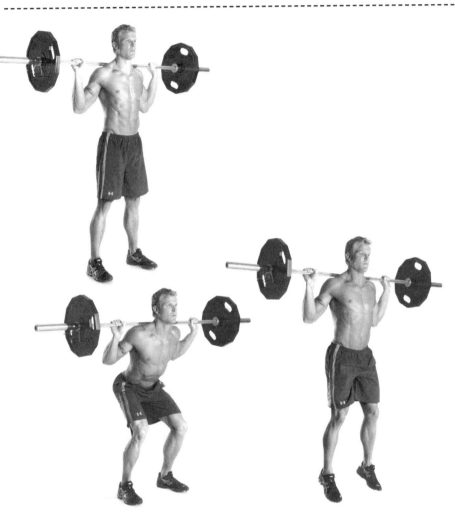

START POSITION

➜ Place a barbell across your upper trapezius and grab the bar with an overhand grip, hands more than shoulder-width apart and feet hip-width apart.

THE MOVE: Quickly bend your knees and squat so that your thighs are at a 45-degree angle from the floor—about half the distance you would dip for a full squat. Immediately push through your heels and jump straight up so that your feet leave the floor. Land on your toes to absorb the impact and immediately repeat the exercise.

OSCAR J QUEZADA

BUTCHER   PALATINE, IL

33
CURRENT AGE

5'7"
HEIGHT

198
STARTING WEIGHT

186
6 WEEKS LATER

RESULTS: Quezada lost 12 pounds and figures he gained a few in muscle weight because his body looks so different. "People, women especially, notice my chest and arms even when I wear baggy clothes. They'll say, 'Have you been working out?'

Quezada boosted his bench press by 15 pounds in the first few weeks of the program. He attributes the strength gains to the program's emphasis on the dead lift and different bench press exercises. He says that the workouts are so exhausting that his insomnia has been relieved significantly. "I used to be a zombie at work. Now, I have a lot of energy."

"People, women especially, notice my chest and arms even when I'm wearing baggy clothes."

A knee injury put an end to Oscar Quezada's running ritual that kept him lean. As a result, he took up another habit: eating cookies. "My eating went to crap," he says. "White bread, pizza, bad carbs. I put on a lot of body fat."

Quezada didn't feel healthy, strong, or particularly energetic. Something was wrong. His insomnia was getting worse and his body looked flabby. Then he saw a Tweet about the Testosterone Transformation workout and decided to take a look at the exercise plan. "It was fresh. I had been bored by weight lifting because it's so repetitive. But this had exercises I'd never done before. I love the tire flipping; it's one of my favorite things to do. The plate lunge was cool. And that torturous barbell complex—oh man, that was nasty. The reps just don't stop!"

A butcher by trade, he wakes up at 6 a.m. for work but started getting up at 5 to hit the gym. He drinks whey protein powder mixed in water on his way to the gym. After exercise he downs a protein shake made with chocolate milk or soy milk for the sugar to replace his energy. At work he fills his belly with oatmeal. You would think that Quezada wouldn't have any trouble hitting his Testosterone Transformation protein requirements, but this butcher is also a vegetarian. "I'm able to eat high protein because I bought different kinds of powered proteins, then I eat up to eight eggs a day and I snack on Greek yogurt and almonds." Dinner is often mashed black beans with grilled vegetables topped with cheese in a tortilla, which delivers more protein. For lunch, he eats salads dressed with avocado oil, which gives him the healthy fats he needs to boost his testosterone.

BONUS CHAPTER

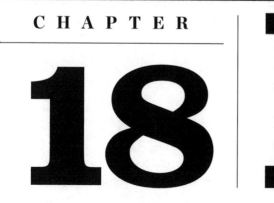

MAXIMUM STRENGTH: THE ADVANCED WORKOUT

Follow the Testosterone Transformation Workout with this ultra-tough 4-week program

CHAPTER

18

If you've completed the Testosterone Transformation Workout, followed our nutrition program, and learned how crucial adequate rest and good sleep are to muscle building, then one thing's for certain: The body you have now is not the body you started with.

But we know what you're thinking. Like the owner of a Ferrari that can go from zero to 100! in just seconds, you're ready to put your newly acquired horsepower into practice. That's why we offer this new master-class workout that will push your strength to the max.

Meet CJ Murphy: CJ Murphy is a certified strength coach and sports nutritionist and owner of Total Performance Sports, in Everett, Massachusetts— a 30,000-square-foot facility that *Men's Health* has recognized as one of America's 20 best gyms.

Murphy is a former strongman competitor and national powerlifting champion and an award-winning trainer who has coached national and world-record powerlifters and North American Strongman competitors. His 20 years of experience have earned him the Spirit of Strength award from USA Master Trainers and the International Sports Sciences Association's (ISSA) Distinguished Achievement Award.

We are privileged to bring you a workout from Murphy that will turbo-boost your T-levels and transform you into a strongman.

Tools For Maximum Strength

Murphy's workout requires a power rack, a pull-up bar, an incline bench, and a barbell—which any good gym will have—plus a few pieces of specialized equipment that you probably won't find at health clubs offering Zumba classes. The hardcore items are a 1½-inch-thick nylon rope, a Manta Ray harness, and a Prowler (also known as a Lung Breaker or a Punisher sled). The names of the equipment alone should make you start sweating.

Finding this stuff may sound like a hassle, but guess what. That's perfect, because it means that you're going to use what few guys know about: the tools that the strongest men on the planet use to build big muscle. With a little digging, you'll find a serious gym filled with serious equipment like this. And if you want to go whole hog and outfit your garage or basement with this gear, check out elitefts.net (for the Prowler and other gear), totalperformances-ports.com (for the LungBreaker, drag sleds and other gear), and GoFit.net (for the training ropes).

However, if you don't have the space or can't find what we recommend at a gym, don't sweat it. We supply alternate exercises that make fair (but not perfect) substitutions so you can still reap some of the results.

The Special Equipment List:

1½-inch-thick, 40- to 50-foot nylon rope: Nylon is ideal because it won't shred from heavy use, plus it's much easier on your hands when you perform the exercise found in this program. This is used for the rope undulation workout called the Battling Rope Tabata on page 319. You can buy the fitness rope online from GoFit.net and other home fitness gear websites. GoFit.net sells its 40-foot Combat Rope for $160.

Manta Ray rear squat support harness: This is a plastic device that clips onto a standard barbell, allowing the lifter to place the bar very high on his back. This pushes the upper back forward forcing the lifter to maintain a hard arch on the upper and lower back. It also takes the stress off of your vertebra by dispersing it evenly across your trapezius. Available from fitness equipment websites and some sporting goods stores.

Prowler or Lung Breaker: This training sled allows you to stack weight plates on top of it so you can either push it forward or pull it backward. If it sounds too cumbersome, consider this: Nothing lets you build muscle and burn fat faster, and it's smaller, lighter, cheaper (average price: $300), and much cooler-looking than a treadmill. Dragging and multi-purpose training sleds start at around $180; various versions of the Prowler are offered from about $280 to $500 from elitefts.net.

YOUR 4-WEEK
MAX-STRENGTH WORKOUT

Murphy's 4-week routine ramps up your T-levels with three separate workouts that focus on improving two specific areas:

▶ **Your limit strength**—the maximum force your muscles can produce in a single contraction. This routine will push those boundaries and raise your limit strength in your legs, your shoulder girdle (through pressing movements), and your back (through pulling movements). "There are many ways to raise limit strength, but for this routine you'll be using a hybrid approach," says Murphy. "For the lower body, you'll focus on heavy-weight, high-volume squatting, but for your upper body, you'll be aiming to hit a 'maximum weight for specific reps' each week."

▶ **Your anaerobic threshold**—the point at which your body's oxygen supply is no longer able to produce enough energy to meet your muscles' demands. Consider this to be your body's energy breaking point—this routine will raise your anaerobic threshold, allowing you to work harder for longer periods.

Using this technique, Murphy's clients get seriously strong and incredibly fit, gain muscle, and lose body fat—all at an alarming rate. "Having a high limit strength makes everything else go up," says Murphy. The higher you can raise your limit strength on the main lifts in this routine—squats, barbell rows, deadlifts, and barbell overhead presses—the more weight you'll be able to handle on the assistance work (the other exercises in Murphy's program).

"The more weight you can handle on the assistance work, the more testosterone you'll have floating around in your system," says Murphy. "You don't need to be a 500-pound bencher or an 800-pound squatter to achieve maximum testosterone—all you need to do is to get as strong as you can for your goals."

That's why Murphy's strength program uses heavy-weight, high-volume squatting, as well as repetition maxes of either 3 or 5 reps on specific lifts. "Training in this fashion will get you stronger and raise your anaerobic threshold while forcing your body to release more testosterone at the same time."

Murphy's Pre-Workout Push

Before you begin each workout, prepare your body with a warmup that consists of three elements: 5 minutes of foam rolling, a few minutes of callisthenics, and a few minutes performing body-weight exercises (the Bodyweight Blitz).

1 Foam Rolling (5 minutes)

"Making your muscles as pliable as possible allows them to contract more efficiently," says Murphy. That's where a simple technique called "self-myo-fascial release" can help. This type of self-administered soft-tissue therapy involves using your own body weight to roll specific body parts back and forth over a piece of round, firm foam. It's a trick that "increases your muscles' range of motion by improving your circulation, loosens up your muscles and connective tissues, and breaks up knots and scar tissue," says Murphy.

All you need is a foam roller, a cylindrical piece of closed-cell foam that you can buy online or find in any sports-medicine, physical-therapy, or sporting-goods store for less than $20. Then spend 5 minutes rolling out all of your major muscle groups. For an idea on how to do it, here are a few examples. To loosen your:

▶ **Glutes:** Sit on the roller and reach your arms behind you for balance. Using your hands for support, slowly roll back and forth and partially from side to side—if you feel any sore or tight spots, pay extra attention to them. These are areas that you need to roll a little longer and harder to break up tissue.

▶ **Hamstrings:** Stay seated and place the roller under your thighs. Slowly roll it up and down your leg from the bottom of your butt toward your knee.

▶ **Calves:** Stay seated and place the roller under your lower legs. Slowly roll up and down from just below your knee down to your ankle.

▶ **Quadriceps:** Lie facedown on top of the roller as if you were doing a pushup (using your hands for balance) and roll it back and forth along the front of the thigh from your hip down to your knee.

▶ **Upper back, trapezius, and rhomboids:** Lie on your back and place the roller underneath your shoulder blades. Bend your knees and place your feet flat on the floor. Pushing off with your feet, run the roller up and down from your head to the middle of your back.

▶ **IT (iliotibial) band** (the band of muscles that runs along the outside of the thigh from hip to knee): Lie on the roller on your left side with the roller placed just below your left hip. Support yourself with your left hand—your right leg should be bent, with your right foot placed in front of you. Roll the roller up and down from your hip down to your knee. Repeat with your right side.

2 Calisthenics

Chaining together a series of 8 to 10 calisthenic exercises into a circuit creates a type of dynamic warmup that accomplishes several things. "It increases your dynamic flexibility [which allows you to move your joints through a full range of motion], it primes your nervous system to fire properly for the training you're about to do, and it raises the body's core temperature to make your muscles warm and pliable so you can lift properly and safely," says Murphy.

Any series of calisthenic exercises can work, such as this example straight from Murphy's own playbook: prisoner squats, jumping jacks, seal hops, straight-leg raises, iron crosses, hip pops, single-leg hip pops, prone cobras, Supermans.

For each exercise, do 8 repetitions, then immediately move to the next exercise, with no rest in between. Perform this type of warmup 2 to 5 times as necessary. "If you're totally gassed after 2 sets, then stop there," says Murphy. "But if you're not warm, then do another."

3 Bodyweight Blitz

Finally, you'll start with a series of three body-weight exercises: back raises (also known as hyperextensions), fat-guy pullups, and regular pushups.

According to Murphy, the reason for performing these exercises prior to your workout is twofold. First, "if you struggle with any of these at the start, then the entire routine is not for you," he says. That means that if this warmup is more like a wear-out for you, wait until you have a little more experience before attempting the routine.

"Two: Adding these exercises increases the time under tension and volume that your muscles experience," says Murphy. "But not to the point that it will interfere with your muscles' recovery, which will ultimately make them stronger in the long haul."

You'll perform each exercise in the order given for a predetermined number of reps before moving on to the next exercise. One thing you'll notice right away is that you'll be asked to do a lot of reps (ranging from 25 to 50). Don't worry, you're not expected to be able to do all of them in one shot. Instead, for each exercise, you'll do as many reps as possible—stopping 1 rep before failure—then rest for as long as it takes to continue or a maximum of 30 seconds, whichever comes first. You'll continue to do this until you achieve the required number of reps.

A) BACK RAISE

This lower-back exercise requires the use of a hyperextension bench, found at most gyms.

START POSITION: Rest the fronts of your thighs on the wide pad and lock your legs underneath the ankle pads. Lock your hands behind your head and bend forward at the waist until your upper body is perpendicular to the floor.

THE MOVE: Initiate the movement by flexing your glutes hard and pushing your hips into the bench. Slowly raise your torso until it's slightly higher than parallel with the floor, then lower yourself back down into the starting position. Repeat.

B) FAT GUY PULLUP

START POSITION: Lie flat on your back inside a power rack with the bar set a few inches higher than arm's length. Your legs should be together and straight. Grab the bar with your hands slightly wider than shoulder-width apart and hang so that your arms are extended. Your body should form a straight line from your head through your feet, with only the edges of your heels touching the floor.

THE MOVE: Holding this position, pull your body up until your chest touches the bar. Pause, lower yourself back down, and repeat.

C) PUSHUP

START POSITION: Place your hands flat on the floor (shoulder-width apart), keeping your arms straight, elbows unlocked. Straighten your legs behind you, drawing your feet together. Rise up on your toes so that the tops of the balls of your feet are touching the floor. Your body should be one straight line from your feet to your head. Finally, apply constant pressure through your hands as if you were trying to turn your thumbs away from your body—doing this activates your lats more and keeps your shoulder blades in the proper position for the move.

THE MOVE: Most men make the mistake of letting gravity take over to lower their chest to the floor. Instead, "pull yourself down with your lats as if you're doing a row," says Murphy. "This will coil more energy into your muscles, making your pushup more effective." Push yourself back up and repeat.

THE MAIN EVENT

Now that your body is prepared for battle, it's time to tackle the workouts that will take your T-levels to heights never experienced before.
The rules of this three-day-a-week routine are simple:

Rule No. 1: Perform each exercise in the order given, resting only for the amount of time indicated. You'll rest for 48 hours between workouts to allow your muscles the time they need to recover.

Rule No. 2: Your top objective is to use as much weight as possible without affecting your form or your technique. "The key is to avoid training to failure," says Murphy. "Leave 1 or 2 reps in the tank in every set. The last rep should be pretty hard, but not extremely difficult—this will prevent you from experiencing adrenal fatigue and allow you to continue to see progress throughout the program."

Rule No. 3: Whenever an exercise progresses from a higher to a lower number of reps on the chart, the repetitions should be handled using a pyramid technique, where you'll add weight after each set. Add just enough weight to keep the number of times you can perform the exercise within the required rep range.

Rule No. 4: Just as you did with the exercises in the Bodyweight Blitz, if you're asked to do a lot of reps for 1 set (from 35 to 55), you're not expected to be able to do all of them in one shot. Instead, do as many reps as possible—stopping 1 or 2 reps before failure—then rest for only as long as it takes to continue or a maximum of 30 seconds, whichever comes first. You'll continue to do this until you achieve the required number of reps.

Rule No. 5: Whenever you see "3RM" or "5RM" in the chart, that means 3-rep max or 5-rep max. Determine the amount of weight that you can lift for only 3 or 5 reps with good form. Prior to doing these lifts, perform a few warmup sets. (See "Warm Up the Right Way," below.) Do no more than 2 or 3 sets of the 3RM and 5 RM lifts.

WARM UP
THE RIGHT WAY

WHEN PERFORMING WARMUP sets for the heavy main lifts—squats, barbell rows, deadlifts, and barbell overhead presses—don't treat them like working sets. "They are only necessary to prepare your body to handle the big weight," says Murphy. That means don't perform too many reps. "Doing too much volume when warming up is one of the most common mistakes men make that will shortchange you by burning you out before you move on to the heavier weight loads that can make the biggest difference."

Here is a good example of a proper squat warmup for someone squatting 300 pounds for 12 reps for the first working set:

(1) Bar x 10 reps for 2 sets

(2) 135 x 5 reps for 1 set

(3) 185 x 3 reps for 1 set

(4) 225 x 1 rep for 1 set

(5) 265 x 1 rep for 1 set

Proceed to first working set at 300. "On any other exercises, there is very little need for a warmup set," says Murphy. "Your body won't get much warmer than it already is after you perform squats or presses." So for any other exercises, simply jump right into your first set.

THE ADVANCED WORKOUT

WARMUP

Begin each day's program with Murphy's Pre-Workout Push: foam rolling, calisthenics,
and the Bodyweight Blitz. Week 1 Blitz: 25 back raises, 25 fat guy pullups, and 25 pushups.

DAY 1

EXERCISE	Rest between sets	REPS	SETS
MANTA RAY SQUAT	180 seconds max	12	3
BARBELL ROW	60 seconds	10–12, 8–10, 5–8	3
BACK EXTENSION	60 seconds	10–12, 8–10, 5–8	3
INCLINE DUMBBELL BENCH PRESS	60 seconds	10–12, 8–10, 5–8	3
WEIGHTED SITUP	60 seconds	5	5
PROWLER SPRINT	60 seconds	100 feet	6

DAY 2

EXERCISE	Rest between sets	REPS	SETS
BARBELL OVERHEAD PRESS	180 seconds max	5RM	2
KEYSTONE DEADLIFT	60 seconds	10–12, 8–10, 5–8	3
PULLUP	N/A	35	1
BARBELL SHRUG	60 seconds	10–12, 8–10, 5–8	3
SINGLE-ARM FARMER'S WALK DEADLIFT	60 seconds	5	3
HEAVY PROWLER PUSH	60 seconds	100 feet	6

DAY 3

EXERCISE	Rest between sets	REPS	SETS
BARBELL ROW	180 seconds max	5RM	2
DEADLIFT	180 seconds max	5	3
SINGLE-ARM DUMBBELL OVERHEAD PRESS	60 seconds	10–12, 8–10, 5–8	3
BARBELL STEP-UP	60 seconds	10–12, 8–10, 5–8	3
HANGING LEG RAISE	N/A	35	1
BATTLING ROPE TABATA	See exercise description	See exercise description	1

THE ADVANCED WORKOUT

WARMUP

Begin each day's program with the Pre-Workout Push. Week 2 Bodyweight Blitz:
35 back raises, 35 fat guy pullups, and 35 pushups.

DAY 1

EXERCISE	Rest between sets	REPS	SETS
MANTA RAY SQUAT *(ADD 10%)*	180 seconds max	15	3
BARBELL ROW	60 seconds	12–15, 10–12, 8–10, 5–8	4
BACK EXTENSION	60 seconds	12–15, 10–12, 8–10, 5–8	4
INCLINE DUMBBELL BENCH PRESS	60 seconds	12–15, 10–12, 8–10, 5–8	4
WEIGHTED SITUP	60 seconds	5	5
PROWLER SPRINT	60 seconds	100 feet	8

DAY 2

EXERCISE	Rest between sets	REPS	SETS
BARBELL OVERHEAD PRESS	180 seconds max	3RM	2–3
KEYSTONE DEADLIFT	60 seconds	12–15, 10–12, 8–10, 5–8	4
PULLUP	n/a	45	1
BARBELL SHRUG	60 seconds	12–15, 10–12, 8–10, 5–8	4
SINGLE-ARM FARMER'S WALK DEADLIFT	60 seconds	5	3
HEAVY PROWLER PUSH	60 seconds	100 feet	6

DAY 3

EXERCISE	Rest between sets	REPS	SETS
BARBELL ROW	180 seconds max	3RM	2–3
DEADLIFT	180 seconds max	5	5
SINGLE-ARM DUMBBELL OVERHEAD PRESS	60 seconds	12–15, 10–12, 8–10, 5–8	4
BARBELL STEP-UP	60 seconds	12–15, 10–12, 8–10, 5–8	4
HANGING LEG RAISE	N/A	45	1
BATTLING ROPE TABATA	See exercise description	See exercise description	1

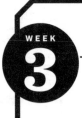

THE ADVANCED WORKOUT

WARMUP

Begin each day's program with the Pre-Workout Push. Week 3 Bodyweight Blitz:
40 back raises, 40 fat guy pullups, and 40 pushups.

DAY 1

EXERCISE	Rest between sets	REPS	SETS
MANTA RAY SQUAT *(ADD 5%)*	180 seconds max	20	1
BARBELL ROW	60 seconds	10–12, 8–10, 5–8	3
BACK EXTENSION	60 seconds	10–12, 8–10, 5–8	3
INCLINE DUMBBELL BENCH PRESS	60 seconds	10–12, 8–10, 5–8	3
WEIGHTED SITUP	60 seconds	5	5

DAY 2

EXERCISE	Rest between sets	REPS	SETS
BARBELL OVERHEAD PRESS	180 seconds max	1RM	2-3
KEYSTONE DEADLIFT	60 seconds	10–12, 8–10, 5–8	3
WEIGHTED PULLUP	N/A	35	1
BARBELL SHRUG	60 seconds	10–12, 8–10, 5–8	3
SINGLE-ARM FARMER'S WALK DEADLIFT	60 seconds	5	3
HEAVY PROWLER PUSH	60 seconds	100 feet	4

DAY 3

EXERCISE	Rest between sets	REPS	SETS
BARBELL ROW	180 seconds max	3RM	2-3
DEADLIFT	180 seconds max	5	5
SINGLE-ARM DUMBBELL OVERHEAD PRESS	60 seconds	10–12, 8–10, 5–8	3
BARBELL STEPUP	60 seconds	10–12, 8–10, 5–8	3
HANGING LEG RAISE	N/A	55	1
BATTLING ROPE TABATA	See exercise description	See exercise description	2

THE ADVANCED WORKOUT

WARMUP

Begin each day's program with the Pre-Workout Push. Week 4 Bodyweight Blitz:
50 back raises, 50 fat guy pullups, and 50 pushups.

DAY 1

EXERCISE	Rest between sets	REPS	SETS
MANTA RAY SQUAT (USE SAME WEIGHT USED DURING WEEK 3)	180 seconds max	12	3
BARBELL ROW	60 seconds	12–15, 10–12, 8–10, 5–8	4
BACK EXTENSION	60 seconds	12–15, 10–12, 8–10, 5–8	4
INCLINE DUMBBELL BENCH PRESS	60 seconds	12–15, 10–12, 8–10, 5–8	4
WEIGHTED SITUP	60 seconds	5	5
PROWLER SPRINTS	See exercise description	100 feet	10

DAY 2

EXERCISE	Rest between sets	REPS	SETS
BARBELL OVERHEAD PRESS	180 seconds max	5RM	2
KEYSTONE DEADLIFT	See exercise description	12–15, 10–12, 8–10, 5–8	4
WEIGHTED PULLUP	N/A	45	1
BARBELL SHRUG	60 seconds	12–15, 10–12, 8–10, 5–8	4
SINGLE-ARM FARMER'S WALK DEADLIFT	See exercise description	5	4
HEAVY PROWLER PUSH	60 seconds	100 feet	3
PROWLER SPRINTS	60 seconds	100 feet	3

DAY 3

EXERCISE	Rest between sets	REPS	SETS
BARBELL ROW	180 seconds max	5RM	2
DEADLIFT	180 seconds max	5	3
SINGLE-ARM DUMBBELL OVERHEAD PRESS	See exercise description	12–15, 10–12, 8–10, 5–8	4
BARBELL STEPUP	60 seconds	12–15, 10–12, 8–10, 5–8	4
HANGING LEG RAISE	N/A	60	1
BATTLING ROPE TABATA	See exercise description	See exercise description	2

BACK EXTENTION

glutes, lower back, core, and hamstrings

START POSITION

➜ Secure your ankles under the foot rollers of a hyperextension bench and rest your upper thighs on the hip pad so that your torso is hanging off the bench. Place your hands behind your head and slowly bend forward at the waist as far as you comfortably can.

THE MOVE: Squeeze your glutes and slowly raise your torso until your upper body is in line with your lower body. Pause for a second or two, slowly lower yourself until the top of your head points to the ground, and repeat.

For this exercise you will need a hyperextension bench

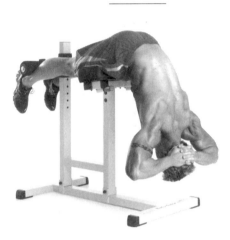

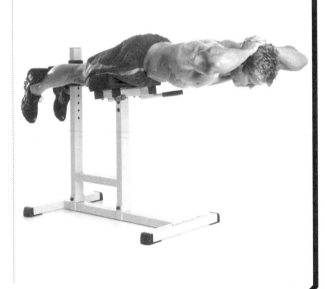

★ TRAINER'S TIP

As you get stronger, try extending your arms out in line with your head, or hold a weight plate with both hands to your chest.

BARBELL OVERHEAD PRESS

MUSCLES TARGETED:
shoulders and triceps

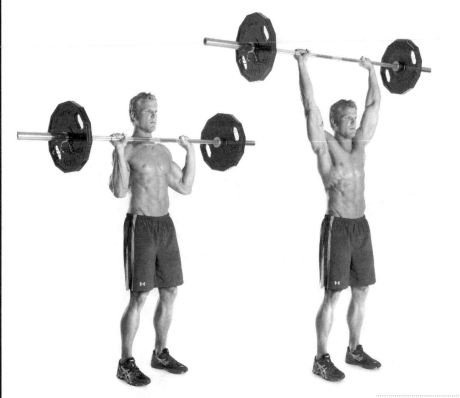

START POSITION

➜ Place a barbell on a rack at about chest-height. With your feet shoulder-width apart, grab the barbell with an overhand grip, take it off the pins, and hold it directly in front of your chest.

THE MOVE: Take a forceful breath in through your mouth to fill your chest up with air, squeeze your glutes as hard as you can, and keep them flexed throughout the entire rep. Now drive the weight overhead—as the bar passes your face, push your head and shoulder girdle forward through your arms and finish with the weight overhead, elbows locked. The bar should be directly over the center of your body. Lower, reset—taking in another breath and squeezing your glutes—and repeat.

★ TRAINER'S TIP

"Try to accelerate the weight as you approach lockout," says Murphy. "If you're doing it correctly, you should hear the weight snap at the top of the movement." Also, do not skip the step of keeping your glutes flexed throughout each rep—this prevents you from using your hips to drive the weight up. "You want to do a strict overhead press using the pressing muscles only," says Murphy.

BARBELL ROW

MUSCLES TARGETED:
latissimus dorsi, middle trapezius, and lower back

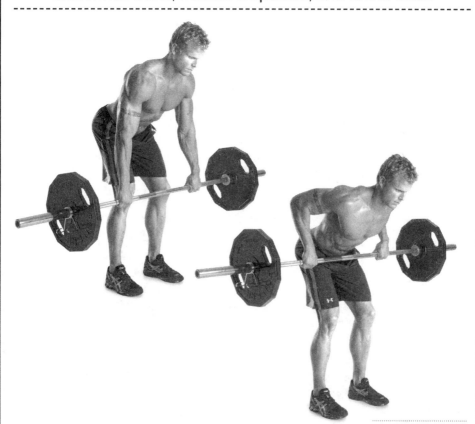

START POSITION

→ Place a barbell in a rack at about knee height. Grab the bar with a shoulder-width overhand grip and stand up straight. Squeeze your shoulder blades together and down and lock them in that position. Push your hips back—holding a tight arch in your upper and lower back—and stop when the bar is just above your kneecaps. Your body should be at a 45-degree angle.

THE MOVE: Row the bar up your thighs and pull it to your lower abdomen. Lower and repeat, keeping the bar in contact with your thighs the entire time. Make sure your shoulder blades are squeezed together and down. "Imagine you're trying to pull your elbows toward your butt as you row," says Murphy.

★ TRAINER'S TIP

Check your body position as the reps pile up. "Most people have a tendency to stand up straight as the set goes on," says Murphy. "Make sure that you stay at a 45-degree angle for the whole set. You can easily do this by shifting your weight toward your heels—and pushing your butt back a little—if you find that you've straightened up a little."

BARBELL SHRUG

MUSCLES TARGETED:
trapezius

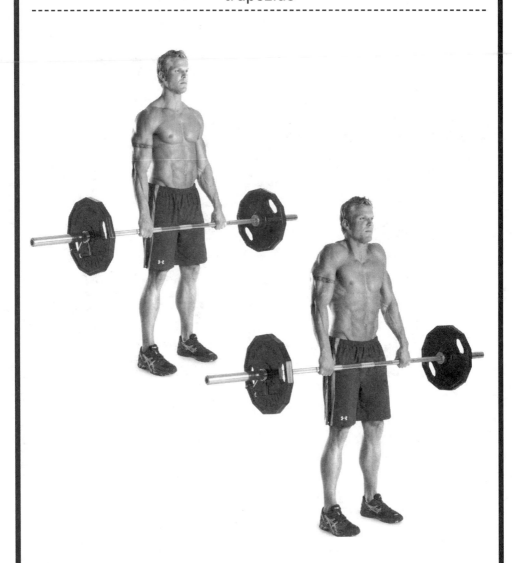

START POSITION

➜ Stand holding a barbell with an overhand grip, with your arms hanging straight down—the bar should be directly in front of your thighs.

THE MOVE: Without bending your arms, raise your shoulders straight up toward your ears as high as you can. Pause for a second, lower the bar back down, and repeat.

BARBELL STEP-UP

MUSCLES TARGETED:
quadriceps, hamstrings, glutes, and calves

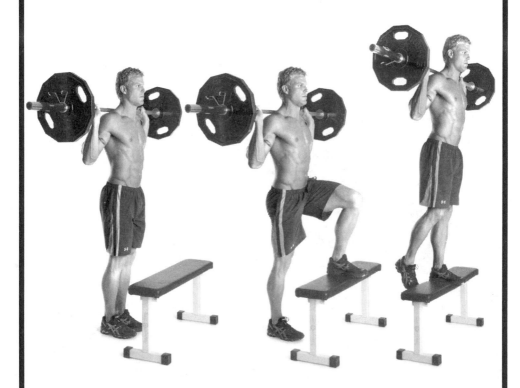

START POSITION

➡ Place a barbell across your upper back and hold it with an overhand grip, palms facing forward. Stand directly in front of a sturdy weight bench with your feet about hip-width apart.

THE MOVE: Arch your back hard, bend your left leg, and place your entire left foot on the bench. Step up onto the bench by driving your left heel into the bench. Pause at the top for a split second, then reverse the motion by stepping back into the start position. Repeat until the desired reps are completed and switch legs.

★ TRAINER'S TIP

"If you're stepping up with your left leg, lift the big toe of your right foot up before you step up," says Murphy. "This will prevent you from cheating by pushing off of your right foot."

BATTLING ROPE TABATA

MUSCLES TARGETED:
chest, arms, forearms, shoulders

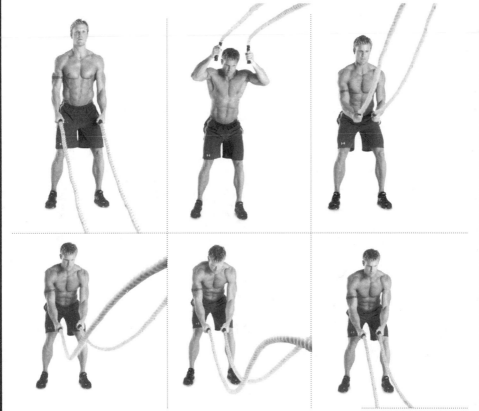

★ TRAINER'S TIP

"Watch the waves that the ropes make," says Murphy. "They should be even and smooth—if one is different from the other, then you need to make sure that you are moving both of your arms evenly." Also, "make sure the waves go all the way to where you have the rope anchored," advises Murphy. "If you're not strong enough to get the waves all the way, shorten the rope by tying a knot in it behind the anchor point."

START POSITION

➜ Wrap the rope evenly around a sturdy object, such as a tree, or thread it around a heavy dumbbell placed flat on the floor. Grab an end in each hand and step back far enough from the anchoring point so that both ends of the rope are straight but not taut. Stand with your feet slightly wider than shoulder-width apart so that you feel as if you have a good center of balance.

THE MOVE: Start moving your arms up and down at the same time as quickly as you can—the rope should begin to create waves in front of you. Do the drill for 20 seconds, then rest for 10 seconds. Repeat 8 times for a total of 4 minutes.

DEADLIFT

trapezius, lower back, hamstrings, and glutes

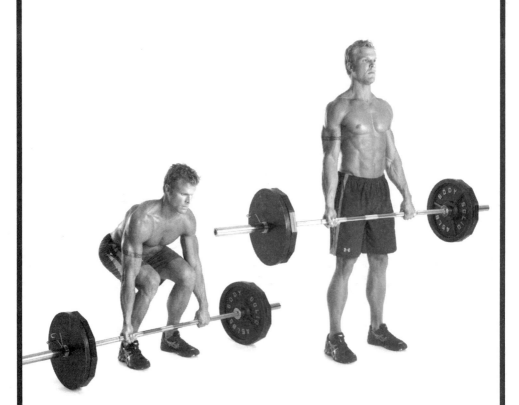

START POSITION

➜ Stand facing a barbell with the bar over your toes, feet hip-width apart. Bend your knees and grasp the bar with an alternating grip (an overhand and underhand grip) and your hands shoulder-width apart.

THE MOVE: Start by squeezing the bar as hard as you can and flexing your lats hard. There should be no slack in your arms before you try to lift the weight, so remove it by lightly pulling the bar up. Once you're set, stand straight up—as the bar passes your knees, drive your hips through by squeezing your glutes hard. Hold at the top of the move for a split second, then lower. Reset your posture and repeat.

★ TRAINER'S TIP

Instead of simply standing up with the weight, imagine that you are pushing the floor away from you through your heels. This mental trick assures that the right muscles are lifting the weight.

HANGING LEG RAISE

MUSCLES TARGETED:
abdominals and core

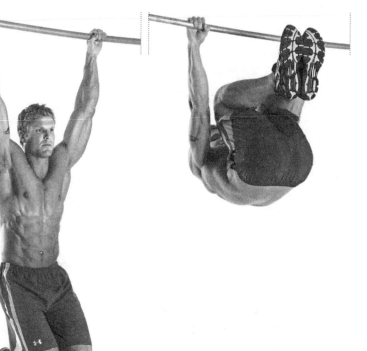

START POSITION

➜ Hang from a chinup bar with your hands spaced more than shoulder-width apart. Your legs should be slightly bent underneath you, with your legs and feet together.

THE MOVE: Keeping your legs and feet together, curl your hips toward your ribs and raise your knees toward your forehead. Pause, lower your legs back down, and repeat.

★ **TRAINER'S TIP**

"Make sure that you drive your knees up as high as you can," says Murphy. "What you're striving for is to get your body curled up into a small, tight ball at the top."

HEAVY PROWLER PUSH

MUSCLES TARGETED:
legs, hips, back, chest, shoulders, and arms

For this exercise, you'll need a Prowler-type weight sled or 45-pound plates.

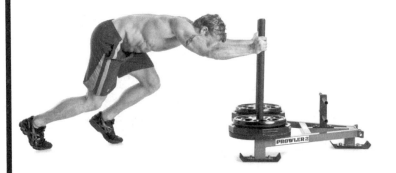

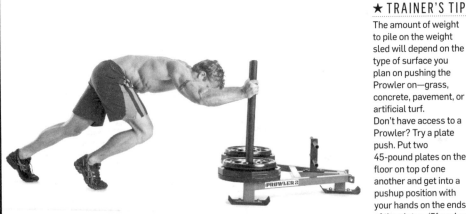

START POSITION

→ Grab the high poles of the Prowler (or the "horns"), extend your arms, and bend forward at the waist.

THE MOVE: Keeping your head down facing the ground, push the sled as hard as you can for the required distance (100 feet)—that counts as one rep. Make sure you're pushing the Prowler on the balls of your feet, driving your force through the floor on one leg for as long as you can before you switch to the other leg.

★ TRAINER'S TIP
The amount of weight to pile on the weight sled will depend on the type of surface you plan on pushing the Prowler on—grass, concrete, pavement, or artificial turf.
Don't have access to a Prowler? Try a plate push. Put two 45-pound plates on the floor on top of one another and get into a pushup position with your hands on the ends of the plates. (If you're on a wooden floor, place the plates on a bath towel doubled over. Drive the plates forward across the floor while maintaining the pushup position, but don't let your butt rise up so that your body looks like an upside-down V as you do it.

INCLINE DUMBBELL BENCH PRESS

MUSCLES TARGETED:
chest, shoulders, and triceps

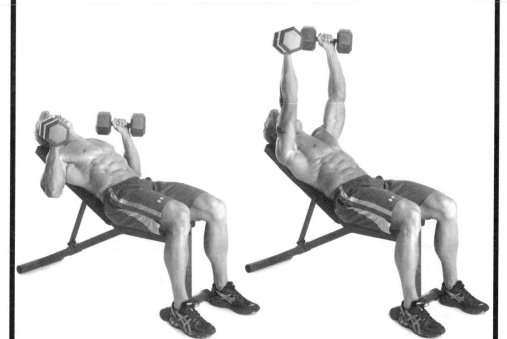

★ TRAINER'S TIP

"Keeping your arms at a 45-degree angle to your body minimizes the damaging force on your rotator cuff muscles, which will benefit you in the long term," says Murphy. Think about "pulling" or rowing the weights down with your lats—don't just lower the dumbbells down, but actively pull them down. This will allow your muscles to store more energy, which will create a stronger press.

START POSITION

➔ Grab a pair of dumbbells and lie back on an incline bench with your legs bent and your feet flat on the floor. Position the weights just outside your chest, with your arms angled at 45 degrees from your body—most guys tend to angle their elbows farther away from their torso, creating a 90-degree angle.

THE MOVE: Press the dumbbells up above your chest until your arms are straight with your elbows in a locked position—your palms should be in a position near 45 degrees to your body. Lower the weights down to the sides of your chest and repeat.

KEYSTONE DEADLIFT

MUSCLES TARGETED:
hamstrings, glutes, and lower back

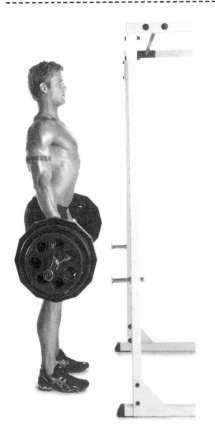 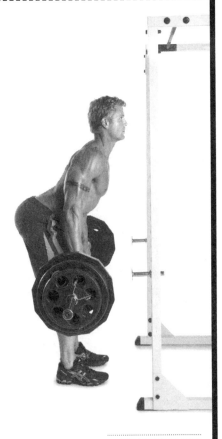

START POSITION

➜ Set a barbell on a power rack at mid-thigh height. Grab it with an overhand shoulder-width grip, step back, then let the bar hang down at arm's length in front of you. Space your feet about hip-width apart. Lift your chest toward the ceiling, push your belly out, and arch your lower back. "This helps if you drive your lats down to the floor as you drive your chest up to the ceiling," advises Murphy. "This locks your posture to do the exercise correctly."

THE MOVE: Begin the movement by pushing your hips back until the bar touches the tops of your knees—it should stay in contact with your legs at all times. Pause, then drive your heels through the floor as you flex your glutes as hard as you can to return to the start position. Reset your posture and repeat.

★ TRAINER'S TIP

"This exercise is a lift that Fred 'Dr. Squat' Hatfield—the first person to squat more than 1,000 pounds—used as a primary assistance exercise to get brutally strong," says Murphy. "It minimizes the force on the lumbar spine if done correctly, allowing you to handle very heavy weight when using good form."

MANTA RAY SQUAT

MUSCLES TARGETED:
quadriceps, hamstrings, glutes, traps, and rhomboids

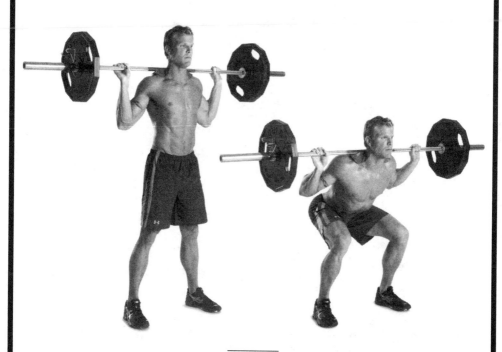

For this exercise, you will need a Manta Ray
(described on page 303)

START POSITION

➜ Place the bar on a squat rack about chest-high and stand in front of it.
Snap the Manta Ray onto the center of the bar. Grab the bar with an
overhand grip slightly wider than shoulder-width apart, duck underneath
it, and rest the bar high across your upper back. Space your feet a little
wider than shoulder width, turning your toes slightly outward.

THE MOVE: Take a deep breath to fill your lungs and push your belly
out. Arch your lower back hard and squeeze your shoulder blades
together and upward—you'll need to keep them in this position for the
entire set. Push your knees out sideways as you sit back, as if you're
sitting on a chair. Stop when your thighs are parallel to the floor, pause
for a second, then stand back up by driving your head and traps into the
bar and pushing through your heels. Repeat. Try to hold your breath for
at least 2 reps as you perform the set.

★ TRAINER'S TIP

Don't have a Manta
Ray? You can opt to do
regular squats (see
page 191).

PROWLER SPRINT

MUSCLES TARGETED:

legs, hips, back, chest, shoulders, and arms

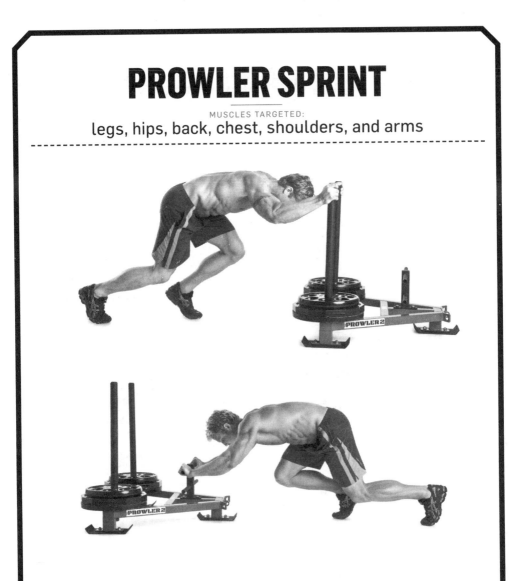

For this exercise, you'll need a Prowler-type weight sled or 45-pound plates.

START POSITION

➜ Grab the high poles of the Prowler (or the "horns"), extend your arms, and bend forward at the waist.

THE MOVE: Keeping your head down facing the ground, push the sled as fast as you can for the required distance (100 feet)—that counts as one rep. Once you reach the 100-foot mark, switch to the opposite side of the Prowler, grab the low handles, and repeat the exercise by pushing it back to your starting point. That's officially 2 reps.

★ TRAINER'S TIP

Do this exercise at a full sprint. Use a weight that allows you to go fast, but not so fast that the Prowler gets ahead of you. If you don't have access to a Prowler, use just a 45-pound plate and try pushing it across the floor as fast as you can.

PULLUP

MUSCLES TARGETED:
latissimus dorsi, rhomboids, lower trapezius, biceps, and forearms

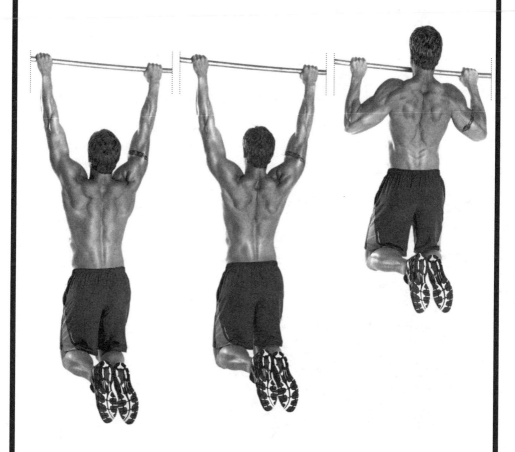

START POSITION

➜ Grab a chin-up bar with an overhand grip, hands shoulder-width apart. Hang from the bar with your arms fully extended.

THE MOVE: Begin by first squeezing your lats and pulling your shoulder blades down. Continue pulling yourself up until your chin is over the bar, hold for a split second, then lower yourself back down until your arms are fully extended. Repeat.

★ TRAINER'S TIP

If you can't do a pullup, loop a Jump Stretch band over the bar, then put one foot on it to stretch it out—the band will assist you through the lift, allowing you to complete the reps.

SINGLE-ARM DUMBBELL OVERHEAD PRESS

MUSCLES TARGETED:
shoulders and triceps

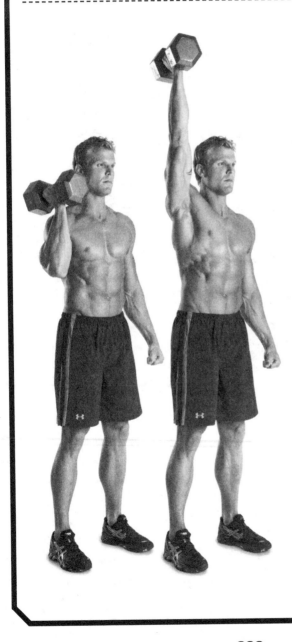

START POSITION
➜ With your feet shoulder-width apart, stand straight, holding a dumbbell in your right hand above shoulder level, with a hammer-style grip (palm facing in).

THE MOVE: Keeping your back straight and eyes staring forward—not up at where the weight will be moving—press the weight up over your head until your arm is straight, elbow locked. Lower the weight, then repeat the exercise. Perform the desired reps and switch positions to work your left side.

★ TRAINER'S TIP
As you press the weight up with one hand, squeeze your other hand as tightly as you can throughout the lift. "This technique creates tension throughout all of your muscles, making your body more stable so you can deliver more force," says Murphy.

SINGLE-ARM FARMER'S WALK DEADLIFT

MUSCLES TARGETED:
total body and core

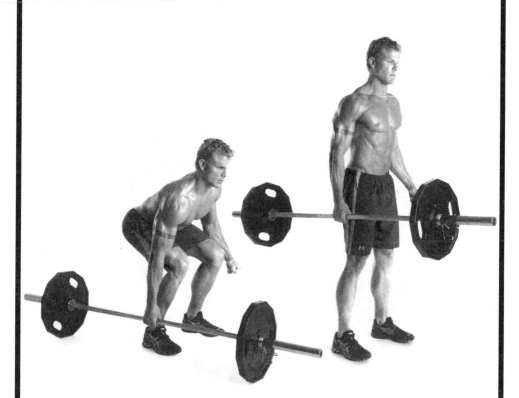

START POSITION

➜ With your feet shoulder-width apart, stand alongside a barbell so that the middle of the bar is next to your right leg. Arch your upper and lower back hard and push your hips back so that your body lowers far enough to grab the bar with your right hand in the center of the bar (palm facing in toward your leg). Finally, take all of the slack out of your arm by slightly pulling on the bar.

THE MOVE: Pushing through your heels, stand straight up, keeping a tight arch throughout your back. Lower the barbell back down to the floor and repeat. Perform the required number of reps, then switch positions to work the opposite side.

★ TRAINER'S TIP

"Try imagining that you have a bar in each hand," says Murphy. "This trick will keep your body from twisting to one side as you perform the lift."

WEIGHTED PULLUP

MUSCLES TARGETED:
latissimus dorsi, rhomboids, lower trapezius, biceps, and forearms

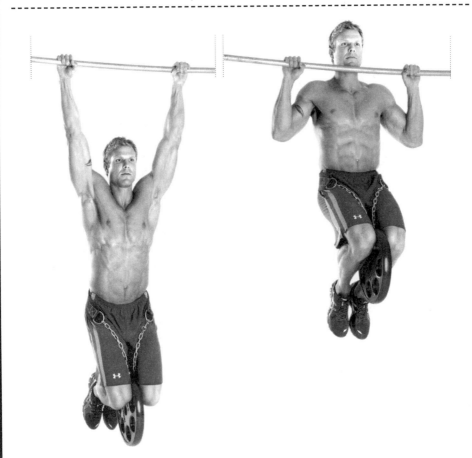

For this exercise, you'll need a weighted vest or a dip belt.
If you don't have one, ask a training partner to place a dumbbell between your legs
just above the knees; brace it there by squeezing your legs together.

START POSITION
➜ Grab a chinup bar with a pronated grip (overhand), hands shoulder-width apart. Hang from the bar with your arms fully extended.

THE MOVE: Begin by first squeezing your lats and pulling your shoulder blades down. Continue pulling yourself up until your chin is over the bar, hold for a split second, then lower yourself back down until your arms are fully extended. Repeat.

WEIGHTED SITUP

MUSCLES TARGETED:
rectus abdominis

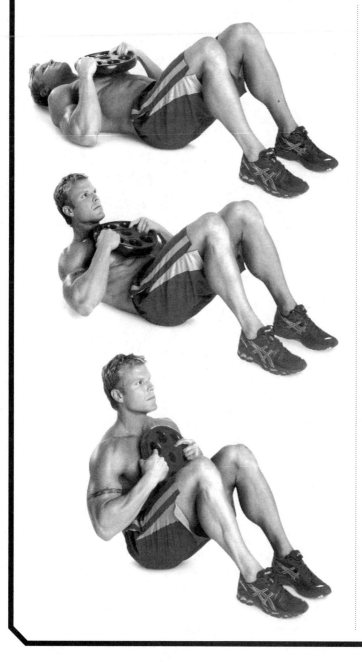

START POSITION

➡ Lie flat on a mat with your knees bent and feet flat on the floor, about shoulder-width apart. Grab a weight plate (2½ to 5 pounds to start) and hold it at your chest with both hands—your elbows should naturally face either out to your sides or straight up. Lift the pelvic floor first by squeezing the same muscles you would use to stop yourself from urinating—you'll keep them contracted for the entire exercise.

THE MOVE: Lift your head and shoulders up off the floor—imagine you're pulling your ribs toward your hips with your abs. As you come up, continue to lift your torso off the floor into a full situp. Lower and repeat.

Index

Boldface page references indicate illustrations or photographs.
Underscored references indicate boxed text.

A

Ab wheel, 116
Ab wheel hand walking, 140, **140**
Adenosine triphosphate (ATP), 273
Adrenal fatigue, 308
Adrenal glands, 8, 13
Adrenaline, 24
Aerobic exercise
    HIIT, 95–96, 129
    testosterone decrease with, 32, 94–95
Aggression, testosterone association with,
    11
Agility, testosterone and, 15–16
Alcohol, effects of, 257, 263
ALL DAY TEST acronym, 259
Alternating forward lunge, 297, **297**
Alternating hammer curl, 288, **288**
Alzheimer's disease, 14–15
Amino acids
    branched-chain amino acids (BCAAs),
        255, 274–75
    essential, 39, 39, 42–43
    glutamine, 275–76
Anabolic steroid use in sports, 264
Anaerobic threshold, improving, 304
Anatomy, muscle, **247**
Androgen deficiency, 4
Androgenic hormones, 7–8, 264. *See also*
    Testosterone
Arnold press, 194, **194**
Aromatase, 3
Arthritis, decrease with fats, 47
Atherosclerosis, 49
ATP, 273

B

Back extension, 314, **314**
Back raise, 307
Balance, 92
Barbell complex, 168–69, **168–69**

Barbell jump squat, 298, **298**
Barbell overhead press, 315, **315**
Barbell rollout, 170, **170**
Barbell row, 316, **316**
Barbell shrug, 317, **317**
Barbell step-up, 318, **318**
Battling rope tabata, 319, **319**
BCAAs, 274–75
Beans, glycemic index of, 59
Beef
    complete protein, 39
    nutrients incomplete protein, 39–40
Belly fat
    loss with MUFA-rich diet, 50
    testosterone decrease with, 3, 31
Bench press, 141, **141**
Benign prostatic hyperplasia, 264, 265
Bent-over barbell row, 221, **221**
Bent-over barbell row (underhand grip),
    284, **284**, 291, **291**
Bicarbonate, 276
Biceps sled curl, 142, **142**
Bisphenol A (BPA), 25–27, 253, 256–57
Blender, 273
Blood pressure, 264
Body mass index (BMI), 20–21, 25
Bodyweight Blitz warmup, 306–8
Bodyweight lunge, 171, **171**
Bone strength, testosterone and, 16
Bottom end drive, 143, **143**
BPA, 25–27, 253, 256–57
Brain
    control of testosterone production, 8–9
    improvement with polyunsaturated fats,
        47
    testosterone benefits for, 14–15
Branched-chain amino acids (BCAAs), 255,
    274–75
Breads, 59, 81
Breakfast, multivitamin at, 272
Breathing, diaphragmatic, 251–52
Bryant, Josh, 89
Bulgarian isometric squat, 172, **172**

C

Caffeine, 277
Calf raise on leg press, 173, **173**
Calisthenics, 306
Calories
    burned with protein in diet, 37, 272
    calculating number needed, 64–66
    in carbohydrate-rich foods, 79–81
    in fat-rich foods, 81
    in protein-rich foods, 76–78
Calves, foam rolling, 305
Cancer, prostate, 264
Carbohydrates, 53–61
    allocating into meals, 72–75
    calculating amount needed daily, 66
    complex, 54–55
    cravings, 55
    digestion, speed of, 37
    foods rich in
        breads, grains, and pasta, 81
        fruits, 79
        vegetables, 80
    glycemic index (GI), 57–61
    simple, 54
    testosterone levels, effect on, 56–57
Cardio, as warmup, 96
Casein
    bedtime consumption of, 41
    digestion, time required for, 41, 272
    as testosterone friendly supplement,
        272–73
Cereals, glycemic index of, 59
Cheat curl, 144, **144**
Chemicals
    endocrine-disrupting, 26–27
    in grooming products, 258–59
    xenoestrogens, 253
Child-rearing, testosterone decrease with,
    257
Chinup, 145, **145**
Cholesterol
    conversion to testosterone, 9
    improvement with polyunsaturated fats,
        47
    increase with testosterone, 264
    saturated fats and, 48
    sources of
        beef, 39
        eggs, 39
        poultry, 40

Close-grip burnout, 195, **195**
Cognitive function, testosterone benefits
    for, 14–15
Combat rope, 303
Compensatory acceleration training, 91
Competition, effect on testosterone, 254
Conjugated linoleic acid (CLA), 39
Core-stabilization exercises, 92
Coronary artery disease, 14
Cortisol
    breathing effect on, 251, 252
    catabolic nature of, 24
    increase with overtraining, 32
    lowering with BCAAs, 275
    sleep effect on, 25, 251
    stress and, 24
Cosmetics, chemicals in, 258–59
Cravings, carbohydrate, 55
Creatine
    in fish, 40
    supplement, 273–74
        benefits of, 273–74
        versions of, 273
        when to take, 274

D

Dairy products
    glycemic index, 59
    protein in, 40, 77
Deadlift, 222, **222**, 320, **320**
Decline bench reverse crunch, 223, **223**
Decline close-grip bench press, 196, **196**
Decline close-grip bench press with
    EZ-curl bar, 197, **197**
Dehydration, 70–71
Delayed-onset muscle soreness, 275
DHA, 40, 48, 274
Diabetes
    increase risk with saturated fats, 48
    obesity link to, 21
    prevalence of, 21
Diamond pushup, 198, **198**
Diaphragmatic breathing, 251–52
Diet
    high-protein, 37–38
    low-calorie, 30
    low-fat, 259
    low-protein, 30–31
    T-Transformation Diet, 30–31, 63–81

F

Hypogonadism, 10, 262, 263, 265
Hypothalamus, 8–9, 265, 266

I

Immune system, boost with
   glutamine, 275
   polyunsaturated fats, 47
Incline dumbbell bench press, 323, **323**
Incline dumbbell curl, 149, **149**
Incline fly, 150, **150**
Incline fly superset max pushup, 151, **151**
Incline I-Y-T, 152, **152–53**
Incline press, 154, **154**
Indole-3-carbinol (I3C), <u>69</u>
Infertility, with long-term testosterone
      supplementation, 264
Insulin
   release boost from leucine, 275
   sugars, effect of, 36, 56
Insulin-like growth factor 1, 274, 276
Insulin resistance, 14
Intensity, workout, 85, 102
Interval training, 95–96, <u>129</u>
Isoflavones, <u>39</u>
Isoleucine, 274–75
Iso prone ab, 155, **155**
IT (iliotibial) band, foam rolling, 305–6

J

JM press, 202, **202**
Juices, glycemic index of, 59

K

Keystone deadlift, 324, **324**

L

Lactic acid, 88, 276
Land mine, 179, **179**
Lateral lunge, 180, **180**
Lateral press, 203, **203**
Lateral raise and hold, 206, **206**
Lateral raise superset, 204–5, **204–5**
Lateral T-raise, 207, **207**

Lavender oil, 23–24
LDL cholesterol, 40, 47, 48
Leg curl, 181, **181**
Leg extension, 182, **182**
Legumes, 41, 43
Leucine, 274–75
Leydig cells, 9, 265
Libido, low, 263
Lifestyle, Testosterone Transformation, 33
Limit strength, improving, 304
Log, workout, <u>103</u>
Lung Breaker training sled, 103–4, 303
Luteinizing hormone (LH), 9

M

Macronutrients
   allocating into meals, 72–75
   carbohydrates, 53–61
   fat, 45–52
   protein, 35–43
Magnesium aspartate, 276–77
Manta Ray rear squat support harness, 303
Manta Ray squat, 325, **325**
Meals, frequency of, 69–70
Meat, as protein-rich food, 76
Medications, testosterone reduction from,
   266
Medicine-ball power-up, 289, **289**
Medicine-ball smash, 228–29, **228–29**
Melatonin, 252
Metabolic syndrome, 21
Metabolism, decrease with age, 4, 23
Microwave, heating food in, <u>253</u>
Mini-band clamshell, 183, **183**
Mixed Martial Arts Workout, 279–98
   Day One, <u>281</u>, 282–89, **282–89**
      alternating hammer curl, 288, **288**
      bent-over barbell row (underhand
         grip), 284, **284**
      front-and-back barbell shoulder
         press, 286, **286**
      medicine-ball power-up, 289, **289**
      overview, <u>281</u>
      Romanian deadlift, 283, **283**
      squat, 282, **282**
      standing triceps extension, 287, **287**
      3-2-1 bench press, 285, **285**
      warmup, <u>281</u>